POCKET

ANTIOXIDANTS

T0160131

"Amitava Dasgupta's well-researched and well-written book, *Prescription or Poison?*, will be of great value to the consumer. Using published articles in medical literature as well as his own research, the author aims to provide 'an unbiased view of the benefits and dangers of herbal remedies.' ... This book is a superb reference tool for a consumer who takes prescription drugs and wants to avoid conflicts with herbs, food, alcohol, and other substances. It is just as valuable for anyone who wants an authoritative overview of the benefits and dangers of herbal remedies." — *Library Journal*

"*Prescription or Poison? The Benefits and Dangers of Herbal Remedies* is a cautionary resource that provides a balanced, evenhanded, and practical overview of available alternative remedies. Though *Prescription or Poison?* adheres strongly to a scientific viewpoint, the emphasis is above all on the safety of remedies—alternative remedies such as supplements, homeopathy, and Ayurvedic medicines are not derided or denounced, but rather carefully evaluated with solid recommendations on their proper use. Accessible to readers of all backgrounds, *Prescription or Poison?* is an absolute must-have for anyone considering the use of alternative remedies for themselves or loved ones." — *Midwest Book Review*

Winner of a 2010 *American Journal of Nursing* Book of the Year award

DEDICATION

Dedicated to the memory of my father,
the late Anil Kumar Dasgupta

Ordering
Trade bookstores in the U.S. and Canada please contact

Publishers Group West
1700 Fourth Street, Berkeley CA 94710
Phone: (800) 788-3123   Fax: (800) 351-5073

For bulk orders please contact
Special Sales
Hunter House Inc., PO Box 2914, Alameda CA 94501-0914
Phone: (510) 899-5041   Fax: (510) 865-4295
E-mail: sales@hunterhouse.com

Individuals can order our books by calling **(800) 266-5592**
or from our website at **www.hunterhouse.com**

POCKET
ANTIOXIDANTS

AMITAVA DASGUPTA, PhD

Hunter House
PUBLISHERS

Hunter House Inc., Publishers
PO Box 2914
Alameda CA 94501-0914

Library of Congress Cataloging-in-Publication Data
Dasgupta, Amitava, 1958-
Pocket antioxidants / Amitava Dasgupta, PhD. — First edition.
pages cm
Includes bibliographical references and index.
ISBN 978-0-89793-635-4 (pbk.)   ISBN 978-0-89793-636-1 (ebook)
1. Antioxidants — Therapeutic use.   2. Antioxidants — Health aspects.
3. Oxidative stress.   I. Title.
RM666.A555D37 2013
613.2'86 — dc23   2012043811

Project Credits

Cover Design: Jinni Fontana	Publicity Coordinator: Martha Scarpati
Book Production: John McKercher	Rights Coordinator: Candace
Developmental Editor: Jude Berman	Groskreutz
Copy Editor: Kelley Blewster	Publisher's Assistant: Kimberly Kim
Indexer: Candace Hyatt	Customer Service Manager:
Managing Editor: Alexandra Mummery	Christina Sverdrup
Acquisitions Coordinator:	Order Fulfillment: Washul Lakdhon
Susan Lyn McCombs	Administrator: Theresa Nelson
Editorial Intern: Tu-Anh Dang-Tran	Computer Support: Peter Eichelberger
Special Sales Manager: Judy Hardin	Publisher: Kiran S. Rana

Printed and bound by Bang Printing, Brainerd, Minnesota
Manufactured in the United States of America

9 8 7 6 5 4 3 2 1   First Edition   13 14 15 16 17

Contents

Preface viii

Acknowledgments x

**1. Oxidative Stress and Antioxidants:
An Overview** 1
  What Are Free Radicals? 2
  Sources of Free Radicals That Cause
    Oxidative Damage 4
  The Body's Antioxidant Defense 10

2. Oxidative Stress and Disease 15
  Oxidative Stress and Cardiovascular
    Diseases (Heart Diseases) 17
  Oxidative Stress and Various Types of Cancer . . 21
  Oxidative Stress and Diabetes 22
  Oxidative Stress in Liver and Kidney Disease . . 23
  Oxidative Stress and Inflammation 25

**3. The Antioxidants in Fruits, Vegetables,
Spices, and Nuts** 27
  The Antioxidants Found in Fruits and Vegetables 28
  Which Foods Are Good Sources
    of Antioxidant Vitamins? 31
  The Antioxidant Rankings of Various
    Foods and the Effects of Cooking 37

vi | POCKET ANTIOXIDANTS

The Recommended Intake of Antioxidants. . . . 42
The Fruits Rich in Antioxidants 44
The Vegetables Rich in Antioxidants 48
The Spices and Herbs Rich in Antioxidants . . . 51
The Nuts Rich in Antioxidants 53
Organic vs. Conventional?. 53
The Antioxidants in Other Foods 55

**4. The Antioxidants in Tea, Coffee,
and Chocolate** 56
The Antioxidants in Tea and Coffee 56
The Health Benefits of Tea 58
The Health Benefits of Coffee 60
How Much Tea or Coffee? 62
The Antioxidants in Chocolate 63
The Health Benefits (and Drawbacks)
of Chocolate 65

**5. The Antioxidants in Red Wine
and Other Alcoholic Beverages** 67
Moderate Drinking Versus Hazardous Drinking . 68
The Health Benefits of Moderate Drinking. . . . 69
Red Wine: Superior to Other
Alcoholic Beverages 71
Alcohol's Effects on Other Fruits 73

**6. Antioxidant Vitamins and Minerals:
To Supplement or Not?** 74
Vitamin C. 75
Beta-Carotene (Precursor to Vitamin A). 77
Vitamin E 79
Selenium 80
RDAs and Tolerable Upper Limits: A Summary. . 81
Do You Need a Vitamin/Mineral Supplement? . . 81

7. Other Antioxidant Supplements 83
   Antioxidant Herbal Supplements 85
   Other (Nonherbal) Antioxidant Supplements . . 89

Conclusion 91

Notes 92

Resources 98

Index 99

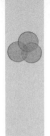

Preface

We have all heard about antioxidants and their importance to health. In fact, the sale of antioxidant vitamins and supplements is a multibillion dollar business that is increasing every year. If you open any health magazine, you will probably see antioxidant supplements advertised as if they were magic bullets, capable of preventing all illnesses by fighting "free radicals." You are probably convinced that free radicals in the body are really bad elements. But did you know that modest amounts of free radicals actually play a vital role in the normal processes of our body? Did you know that scavenging all free radicals by taking in too many antioxidant supplements can cause more harm than good? In fact, if you are healthy, and eat a balanced diet every day that includes generous servings of fruits and vegetables, you will take in enough antioxidants to defend your body from free radicals, and you do not need any supplements.

The purpose of this book is to deliver current medical-level knowledge about the role of antioxidants to consumers in simple, jargon-free language. All important statements and advice in this book are backed by medical research. Each chapter contains carefully cited references. I use my expertise in antioxidant research to interpret and explain complex scientific data in a way that anyone can understand, even readers without a medical background.

I wrote this book because I want to empower you with real scientific data, not myth. My greatest reward for writing this book will be if you, as a reader, use it to find better health.

— Amitava Dasgupta
Houston, Texas

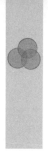

Acknowledgments

I want to thank my wife, Alice, for putting up with the long evening and weekend hours I spent writing this book.

Oxidative Stress and Antioxidants: An Overview

Oxygen is essential for life, but as the body processes oxygen, harmful free radicals are generated as a side effect. Fortunately, substances known as antioxidants can neutralize these free radicals. For healthy living, a delicate balance must be maintained between *oxidative stress* — the damage caused by free radicals — and the body's *antioxidant defense*. If the body's antioxidant defense is not working well, free radicals can produce too much oxidative stress and cause disease.

Oxidation is what we call a chemical reaction in which an oxygen molecule is added to a chemical compound. The most common example of oxidation is the rusting of iron. Another example occurs after cutting an apple and allowing it to sit at room temperature; a brown color will develop due to oxidation. When a compound is oxidized, it exists in what is called an "oxidized state." The opposite chemical reaction, the removal of an oxygen molecule from a chemical compound, is called *reduction*. When a compound is reduced, it exists in what is called "redox state." In general, the cells of our body prefer to exist in a redox state — without any added oxygen.

What Are Free Radicals?

To explain what a free radical is, we have to revisit Chemistry 101. Everything is made up of atoms, which contain smaller parts called protons, neutrons, and electrons. Atoms combine to form molecules, and molecules combine to form chemical compounds. One of the main things that determines how an atom will combine or "bond" with other atoms to form chemical compounds is the number of electrons it contains. If a substance has unpaired electrons, it is unstable or reactive, meaning it is eager to "steal" electrons from another substance so it can become more stable.

A free radical is a highly reactive chemical possessing one or more unpaired electrons. Sometimes a free radical exists for only a fraction of a second or a few seconds before it begins snatching electrons from nearby molecules, thereby changing its chemical structure. It is "free" because it floats around until it stabilizes, and "radical" in the sense that it can steal electrons from a wide variety of molecules.

Above, we defined oxidation as a chemical reaction in which an oxygen molecule is added to a chemical compound. To use the more technical language of chemistry, oxidation is the transfer of one or more electrons from one atom to another. This is important to know, because that's what free radicals do: they "steal" electrons, adding to their own electron count. That means they're involved in the process of oxidation.

Why is this a problem? A free radical will readily react with any molecule in its vicinity, thus damaging that molecule. Let's say the molecule whose electron was stolen by a free radical is part of a bodily tissue. Now that it's missing an electron it has itself become a free radical, on the hunt for electrons to steal. You can see how this ongoing theft of electrons between substances can snowball into a process that wreaks havoc on bodily tissues, leading to disease and premature aging. This harmful state of affairs is called *oxidative stress*.

Here is a list of some of the substances that are vulnerable to damage by free radicals:

- amino acids, the building blocks of all proteins
- carbohydrates, which are utilized by the body for energy
- lipids (fats), including lipids found in cell membranes
- nucleic acids (DNA and RNA), which are present in every cell (except red blood cells) and are responsible for passing on genetic information
- polyunsaturated fatty acids, which are highly concentrated in the brain, where they appear to aid in cognitive and behavioral functioning

On the other hand, small amounts of free radicals are needed for some biological functions. Free radicals:

- activate enzymes that regulate gene function
- help cells communicate with their environment for optimal function
- help with cell division

- help with cell growth and cell proliferation
- regulate immune function
- regulate the redox balance (oxidation–reduction state) of the cell

> **Our body's immune system deliberately generates free radicals to kill invading organisms such as bacteria or viruses.**

As you can see, not all of the effects of free radicals are bad. In addition to the normal processes listed above, strenuous exercise increases the activity of free radicals, but the human body can easily handle this additional oxidative stress.

Sources of Free Radicals That Cause Oxidative Damage

Free radicals come from:

1. internal bodily processes such as infection or inflammation, the body's response to emotional/psychological stress, and normal bodily processes like breathing and processing cellular waste

2. sources external to the body such as environmental and industrial pollutants, some drugs, and radiation

Tables 1.1, 1.2, and 1.3 summarize some of the most significant sources of oxidative stress.

TABLE 1.1. Major Sources of Oxidative Stress

SOURCE	COMMENTS
Air in some industrial environments	Ingestion of mineral particles from dust in individuals working in industry may cause oxidative stress, particularly if the air contains fine metal dust or mineral dust (quartz, silica, asbestos).
Air pollution (e.g., car exhaust)	Exposure to small particles in polluted air can produce significant oxidative stress, increasing risk of asthma, cardiovascular disease, chronic obstructive pulmonary disease (COPD), and lung cancer.
Emotional/psychological stress, depression, anxiety, long-term grief	Psychological stress causes the adrenal glands to secrete "stress hormones" (e.g., cortisol), which are responsible for many reactions, including increased oxidative damage. The effects of short-term stress fade, but chronic stress is linked to many diseases.
Industrial solvents	Some industrial solvents (e.g., benzene, carbon tetrachloride, chloroform, toluene, trichloroethylene, and xylene) may cause oxidative damage if their vapors are inhaled. Some are also carcinogenic (cause cancer). Plant workers may be vulnerable to exposure.
Some household chemicals	See Table 1.2.
Some medications and illicit drugs	See Table 1.3.

(cont'd.)

TABLE 1.1. Major Sources of Oxidative Stress (cont'd.)

SOURCE	COMMENTS
Sunlight and other forms of radiation	Ultraviolet (UV) light contained in sunlight is essential for vitamin D production in the body, but too much exposure can cause sunburn, skin problems, cataracts, and skin cancer. X rays and other forms of radiation can cause oxidative stress. Radiation from airport security screening is too low to be at all unsafe, but radiation therapy used in treating cancer induces oxidative stress due to the intensity of radiation.
Tobacco smoking and secondhand tobacco smoke	Cigarette smoking is the leading cause of preventable death in the United States. Oxidants present in tobacco smoke can damage lungs, causing COPD, chronic bronchitis, and even lung cancer. Smoking also increases risk for atherosclerosis (thickening of the coronary arteries); cancers of the throat, mouth, stomach, and bladder; and asthma (especially in children breathing secondhand smoke).

Not all household chemicals contain the potentially harmful active ingredients listed in Table 1.2 on the next page. Using nontoxic or "earth-friendly" cleaners and personal-care products (body soap, shampoo, etc.) is a good way to reduce your exposure to oxidative stress in the home.

TABLE 1.2. Household Chemicals That May Induce Oxidative Stress

HOUSEHOLD CHEMICAL	ACTIVE INGREDIENT	TOXICITY
IN THE KITCHEN		
All-purpose cleaners	Ammonia, phosphate	Very toxic
Dishwashing detergent	Phosphate	Fairly safe
Oven cleaners	Lye (sodium/potassium hydroxide)	Very toxic
Window/glass cleaner	Ammonia and isopropanol	Very toxic
IN THE LAUNDRY ROOM		
Bleach	Sodium hypochlorite	Moderate
Insect repellent	Organophosphorus or carbamate	Toxic
Laundry detergent	Cationic or anionic substance	Fairly safe
IN THE BATHROOM		
Drain cleaner	Lye or sulfuric acid	Very toxic
Mold removers	Chlorine/ammonium chloride	Toxic
Nail polish remover	Acetone	Moderate
Toilet bowl cleaner	Strong acid or acid + surfactant	Very toxic
IN THE LIVING ROOM		
Air freshener	Formaldehyde, petroleum distillate, para-dichloro-benzene, aerosol propellants	Toxic if ingested
Furniture polish	Ammonia, phenol nitrobenzene, phenol, petroleum distillate	Toxic
Rug/carpet cleaners	Naphthalene + perchloro-ethylene	Toxic fumes

(cont'd.)

TABLE 1.2. Household Chemicals That May Induce Oxidative Stress (cont'd.)

HOUSEHOLD CHEMICAL	ACTIVE INGREDIENT	TOXICITY
IN THE BEDROOM		
Mothballs	Naphthalene	Fairly safe
Spot and grease remover	Chlorinated hydrocarbon	Toxic
IN THE GARAGE		
Antifreeze	Ethylene glycol	Very toxic
Battery	Sulfuric acid and lead	Very toxic if leaking
Motor oil	Complex hydrocarbon, metal	Toxic
Paint/Paint thinner	Toluene	Toxic
Windshield washer	Methanol	Very toxic
IN THE BACKYARD		
Insect repellents	Insecticides	Very toxic
Rodent killer	Warfarin or super warfarin	Very toxic
Swimming pool cleaner	Chlorine, strong acid, hypochlorite	Very toxic
Swimming pool tablet	Sodium or calcium hypochlorite	Toxic (do not drink pool water)
IN THE OFFICE/COMPUTER ROOM		
Glue, rubber cement	Hexane	Moderate
Permanent marker	Xylene	Toxic
Typewriter correction fluid	Acetone	Moderate

During house cleaning or gardening, wear a pair of gloves and a face mask to reduce direct exposure to any household chemicals or volatile organic compounds present in household products.

Common drugs that are also oxidants are listed in Table 1.3 below. Although most people taking these drugs under medical supervision should not have any problems, individuals with glucose 6-phosphate deficiency (a genetic disorder that affects black and Mediterranean people more than Caucasians) may be at much higher risk of oxidative stress from some of them. Glucose 6-phosphate deficiency causes premature destruction of red blood cells, which may be triggered by certain drugs, certain foods (such as fava beans), infection, and severe stress.

TABLE 1.3. Drugs That May Induce Oxidative Stress

TYPE OF DRUG	INDIVIDUAL DRUG
Antibiotics	Bactrim (sulfamethoxazole and trimethoprim), chloramphenicol, ciprofloxacin, moxifloxacin, nalidixic acid, norfloxacin, ofloxacin, sulfacetamide, sulfadiazine, sulfafurazole, sulfanilamide, sulfasalazine
Anticancer drugs	Adriamycin, bleomycin, doxorubicin, menadione, methotrexate, topoisomerase inhibitors
Antimalarial drugs	Chloroquine, mefloquine, pamaquine, primaquine

(cont'd.)

TABLE 1.3. Drugs That May Induce Oxidative Stress (cont'd.)

TYPE OF DRUG	INDIVIDUAL DRUG
Antiretroviral agents	Atazanavir, azidothymidine (AZT), indinavir
Antituberculosis drugs	Dapsone, para-aminosalicylic acid
Diuretics	Spironolactone
Illicit drugs	Cocaine, MDMA (ecstasy)
Immunosuppressants	Cyclosporine A, mycophenolic acid, sirolimus, tacrolimus
Other agents	Ethyl alcohol (alcohol)
Pain relievers	Aspirin, phenacetin

You probably noticed alcohol on the list under "other agents." Drinking alcoholic beverages to excess can induce oxidative stress and cause other serious health problems. On the other hand, drinking alcohol in moderation actually affords many health benefits, and the small amount of oxidative stress induced by moderate amounts of alcohol can be easily counteracted by the body's antioxidant defense mechanism (see Chapter 5).

The Body's Antioxidant Defense

The above tables list lots of potentially harmful agents! How can we possibly counteract all the oxidative stress we're exposed to every day? That's where antioxidants enter the picture.

Antioxidants are substances that neutralize, or counteract, the oxidative stress caused by free radicals. Like free radicals, antioxidants either are produced by the body (*endogenous*) or come from outside the body (*exogenous*, such as the antioxidants found in foods and supplements). Endogenous antioxidants are more powerful than the ones you can get from diet.

The human body makes five types of endogenous antioxidants:

- superoxide dismutase, or SOD
- catalase
- glutathione
- alpha-lipoic acid, or ALA
- coenzyme Q10, or CoQ10

Of these, SOD, catalase, and glutathione provide the highest levels of antioxidant defense.

While it's informative for you to know the names of some of the important endogenous antioxidants, the primary topic of this book is to discuss how you can maximize your intake of exogenous antioxidants by improving your diet. Some common exogenous antioxidants are:

- vitamin A (retinol)
- vitamin C (ascorbic acid)
- vitamin E (alpha-tocopherol)
- selenium (technically a mineral rather than an antioxidant nutrient, but it is a component of antioxidant enzymes)
- beta-carotene (a precursor to vitamin A, meaning it can be converted by the body into vitamin A)
- lutein
- lycopene

Beta-carotene, lutein, and lycopene are all part of the group of plant pigments known as carotenoids. Unlike beta-carotene, lutein and lycopene cannot be converted to vitamin A.

All of these important exogenous antioxidants can be obtained through a healthy, balanced diet. They come mostly from fruits and vegetables. We'll discuss good food sources for them in Chapter 3. Although there are other antioxidants that can be obtained through nutrition, the ones listed above are among the most common.

The focus of this book is to inform you how to maximize your intake of health-promoting antioxidants through diet.

How do we know which fruits and vegetables are high in antioxidants? There are various ways of measuring the antioxidant capacity of foods and supplements, but one of the most common approaches is called the ORAC (oxygen radical absorbance capacity) test. It was developed by scientists at the National Institutes of Health and modified by scientists at the USDA (United States Department of Agriculture). While the exact relationship between the ORAC rating of a food and its health benefits has not been established, foods higher on the ORAC scale are thought to be richer in antioxidant components.

The USDA used to publish the ORAC values of

many foods, spices, and beverages on its website; however, in July 2012 they removed the listing. The reasons they gave were twofold. First, as stated on the website, "ORAC values are routinely misused by food and dietary supplement manufacturing companies to promote their products and by consumers to guide their food and dietary supplement choices." Second, "The values indicating antioxidant capacity have no relevance to the effects of specific bioactive compounds, including polyphenols, on human health."[1]

While most experts agree with the USDA that ORAC values were being misused by food and supplement companies to market their foods, not all agree with the department's second reason for abandoning ORAC values. And certainly not all agree that the USDA should entirely reject ORAC values. To quote Ronald Prior, PhD, a professor in the Department of Food Science at the University of Arkansas, and just one scientist who disagrees with the USDA's decision regarding ORAC scores, "It is unfortunate but true that numbers obtained from ORAC analysis have sometimes been misused, but that does not necessarily mean that the information is not useful if used appropriately."[2]

This book lists the ORAC values of many foods in Chapter 3. It is important for you to be aware that the governmental entity that developed these standards no longer stands by them — not necessarily because the values themselves are incorrect, but because there's some disagreement about how best to use the information.

Certain experts believe, however, that ORAC values still hold merit. That's why I've included them in this book.

Scientists can directly measure various markers in human blood (or urine or bodily tissue) that indicate oxidative stress. In addition, antioxidant compounds such as vitamin C, vitamin E, beta-carotene, and glutathione can be directly measured in the blood to evaluate the antioxidant capacity of the blood. The total antioxidant capacity of the blood is a popular test that a physician can order.

The next chapter outlines diseases that are linked to oxidative stress. After that, we get into the solution: foods and beverages that are rich in antioxidants.

Oxidative Stress and Disease

2

Prolonged oxidative stress has been linked to more than fifty diseases, but evidence of oxidative stress is usually detectable before the onset of disease. The following is a list of most of the common diseases linked to oxidative stress:

- alcohol and drug abuse disorder (abuse of alcohol, amphetamine, nicotine, opioid, hallucinogens)
- alcoholic liver disease
- Alzheimer's disease
- asthma
- attention deficit disorder
- autism
- beta-thalassemia
- bipolar disorder
- cardiovascular disease (heart disease)
- cancers
- chronic depression
- chronic fatigue syndrome
- chronic obstructive pulmonary disease (COPD)
- chronic obstructive sleep apnea
- conditions associated with aging

- convulsions (seizures)
- Crohn's disease
- cystic fibrosis
- diabetes
- delirium
- dementia
- eye diseases (cataract formation, macular degeneration)
- fibromyalgia
- hepatitis and liver diseases
- inflammatatory conditions, including rheumatoid arthritis
- insomnia
- kidney disease
- menopausal symptoms
- obesity and metabolic syndrome
- Parkinson's disease
- phenylketonuria
- psychological and psychosocial stress
- skin disease
- stroke
- sterility and infertility
- transplantation of organs

As discussed in Chapter 1, free radicals are very reactive and can damage many bio-molecules. Cell membranes, which contain lipids, are vulnerable to damage by free radicals, as are proteins. Even DNA, normally a very stable molecule, can be damaged by free radicals, potentially leading to genetic mutation, cancer, aging, and even cell death.

Free radicals can damage virtually all molecules, including carbohydrates, lipids, proteins, and even very stable DNA.

This chapter takes a closer look at the links between oxidative stress and heart disease, certain cancers, diabetes, liver and kidney disease, and inflammatory conditions.

Oxidative Stress and Cardiovascular Diseases (Heart Diseases)

Cardiovascular disease is the number-one killer in the United States. In general, cardiovascular diseases can be broadly classified into two categories:

1. diseases of blood vessels that supply blood to the heart
2. diseases of the heart itself, including congenital defects (birth defects)

Disease of the blood vessels causes heart attack (myocardial infarction). This occurs when plaque builds up in the vessels, narrowing the arteries that supply blood to the heart. When blood flow to the heart is completely blocked, heart attack occurs. Oxidative stress encourages plaque formation because oxidized lipids deposit on arterial walls much faster than unoxidized lipids.

You've probably heard of low density lipoprotein (LDL, aka bad cholesterol). It has been generally accepted that oxidized LDL cholesterol plays an important role in the development of plaque inside arterial walls.

Heart disease has both uncontrollable and controllable risk factors. The uncontrollable risk factors are as follows:

- age (men over 55 and postmenopausal women are at higher risk)
- chronic kidney disease (a risk of heart attack is also high after a kidney transplant)
- family history of heart disease
- sex (males are at higher risk)
- race (African Americans, Hispanics, and American Indians are at higher risk)

The controllable risk factors are as follows (the ones in italics overlap with disease conditions commonly associated with oxidative stress):

- abnormal lipid profile (blood levels of cholesterol and triglycerides)
- *diabetes* (controlling blood sugar is vital to reducing risk)
- high C-reactive protein in blood
- high homocysteine level in blood
- *high level of uncontrolled stress/anxiety/anger*
- hypertension (high blood pressure, which must be controlled by medication and exercise)
- *illegal drug use* (e.g., amphetamines, cocaine, marijuana)

- *obesity* (more than 20 percent over ideal body weight)
- physical inactivity
- poor diet (see Table 2.1)
- *prolonged untreated depression*
- *smoking*

> **Many of the controllable risk factors for heart disease overlap with diseases linked to prolonged oxidative stress.**

Table 2.1 provides a quick summary of how diet can increase or decrease your risk for heart disease.

TABLE 2.1. How Your Diet Affects Your Risk for Heart Disease

Diet contributing to a decreased risk	• Consume plenty of fruits and vegetables every day. In particular, eat blackberries, blueberries, strawberries, and other berry fruits high in antioxidants (see Chapter 3). • Eat 2–3 servings of fish each week. • Eat tree nuts, e.g., hazelnuts, pecans, pistachio nuts, walnuts.
Diet contributing to an increased risk	• Fried foods, including fast foods. • Salty snacks. • Consumption of red meat on a regular basis; regular consumption of animal fat.

Quite a bit of scientific evidence establishes the importance of diet in heart health. Just a couple of studies are summarized here. In one study involving 313,074 men and women without a previous history of heart attack, the authors demonstrated that eight servings of fruits and vegetables (80 grams of fruit and 80 grams of vegetables) a day can significantly lower the risk of heart attack.[1] Eating fish at least twice a week has been shown to reduce the risk of death from sudden heart attack by up to 50 percent.[2] Pregnant women, women planning to become pregnant, and children should not eat certain predator fish, including shark, swordfish, king mackerel, golden bass, and golden snapper, whose flesh can store high amounts of mercury. People who aren't in these risk groups can eat up to seven ounces of these varieties of fish per week. Salmon, cod, flounder, catfish, and other seafood such as crabs and scallops may also contain mercury but in much lower amounts.

Eating fruits and vegetables can provide enough antioxidant defense to lower the risk of heart attack.

Emotion can also affect heart health. As mentioned in Chapter 1, anxiety and depression can produce oxidative stress. Emotionally stressful events, in particular episodes of anger, are capable of triggering the onset of acute heart attack.

Oxidative stress may also be indirectly related to other heart diseases, including:

- arrhythmia (abnormal heart beat)
- cardiomyopathy (disease involving the heart muscle itself)

- congestive heart failure (in which the heart is not pumping blood to its full capacity)
- problems with heart valves
- some congenital heart diseases (birth defects) involving the structure of the heart or of the blood vessels supplying blood to the heart

Oxidative Stress and Various Types of Cancer

The relationship between oxidative stress and cancer is complex. As mentioned earlier, oxidative stress can damage a cell's DNA, causing it to mutate, which in turn may cause tumor cells to form. In addition, oxidative stress can interfere with the communication between cells that governs proper physiological functioning, another condition that can lead to abnormal cell growth, resulting in tumor formation. A simple diagram illustrating the relationship between oxidative stress and cancer appears in Figure 2.1.

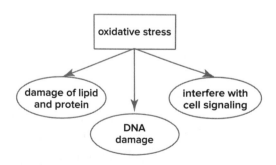

Figure 2.1. How oxidative stress causes cancer

It has been speculated that almost all cancer cells produce more oxygen free radicals than normal cells.[3] Current research indicates that oxidative stress is associated with many types of cancer, including the following:

- bladder cancer
- breast cancer
- colon and rectal cancer
- kidney cancer (renal cell carcinoma)
- liver cancer
- leukemia (blood cancer)
- lung cancer
- oral cancer
- melanoma (skin cancer)
- ovarian cancer
- pancreatic cancer
- prostate cancer
- thyroid cancer

Oxidative Stress and Diabetes

There are two types of diabetes. In *type 1 diabetes*, also called juvenile diabetes, the body produces no insulin. (Insulin is the hormone that regulates blood sugar levels by allowing the cells to utilize this sugar, called glucose, for energy.) Type 1 diabetes usually has its onset in childhood and must be treated with insulin injections. In *type 2 diabetes*, the more common type, the body produces insulin, but the tissues of the body have become "resistant" to insulin — meaning insulin can't do its job of regulating blood glucose levels. Type 2 diabetes usually occurs in adults older than forty (although earlier onset is possible) and can typically be treated with oral medications and changes in diet and exercise habits. Whereas type 1 diabetes is a congenital (genetic) disease caused by the body's reaction against its own insulin-producing cells, type 2 diabetes is generally caused by poor lifestyle (although some people may have a genetic predisposition to type 2 diabetes, even if they follow a healthy lifestyle). Both types of diabetes, if left untreated, have as their main symptom elevated blood glucose levels, called hyperglycemia.

> **Prolonged oxidative stress can increase risk for type 2 diabetes.**

In type 2 diabetes, the cells in the pancreas that normally produce insulin (beta cells) may be damaged by oxidative stress. In addition, oxidative stress can lead to insulin resistance in muscle and liver tissues, where insulin normally helps to break down glucose. Both hyperglycemia and added oxidative stress can cause complications of diabetes (see Figure 2.2 on the following page).

Oxidative Stress in Liver and Kidney Disease

The liver is the major organ that detoxifies the body of drugs and other chemicals. Free radicals are generated

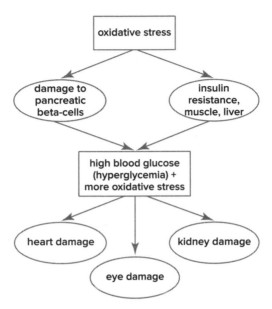

Figure 2.2. How oxidative stress causes type 2 diabetes and worsens its complications

during the normal functioning of the liver. However, certain substances, such as alcohol and some drugs, can cause greater oxidative stress to the liver than normal.

Certain drugs, for example the common pain reliever acetaminophen (the active ingredient in Tylenol and many other medications), can generate free radicals while they're being metabolized in the liver.

Oxidative stress has been linked to the following liver diseases:

- hepatitis (inflammation of the liver)
- alcoholic liver disease
- nonalcoholic liver disease, e.g., fatty liver disease

Furthermore, oxidative stress has been demonstrated in chronic kidney disease and in hemodialysis patients.

Oxidative Stress and Inflammation

Oxidative stress is linked to various diseases involving inflammation. Inflammation is a response of a tissue to injury, which is often caused by an invading microorganism. It is characterized by:

- increased blood flow to the tissue
- increased immune function to destroy the invading organism
- increased production of free radicals in inflamed tissue
- increased temperature
- redness
- swelling
- pain

Inflammation can be acute (short-term) or chronic (long-term). Chronic inflammation is linked to various diseases. Disease names ending with "-itis" (e.g., arthritis, appendicitis, gastritis, laryngitis, pancreatitis, dermatitis, meningitis) are all related to inflammation. In addition, chronic inflammation is linked to asthma, pneumonia, heart disease, diabetes, cancer, Alzheimer's disease, and other illnesses. Once again, you can see how several of these diseases overlap with the illnesses listed at the beginning of the chapter as being related to oxidative stress. Specifically, oxidative stress has been proposed as a factor in Crohn's disease and ulcerative colitis, as well as rheumatoid arthritis — all of which are linked to chronic inflammation.

As this chapter shows, oxidative stress is linked to many diseases. But there's hope. Eating a balanced diet rich in fruits and vegetables is the best way to combat oxidative stress. That's the topic of the next chapter.

The Antioxidants in Fruits, Vegetables, Spices, and Nuts

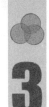

3

The USDA (U.S. Department of Agriculture) recommends that Americans eat a minimum of five servings of fruits and vegetables each day. Fruits and vegetables are our main dietary sources of antioxidants. A wealth of scientific evidence exists showing the potential health benefits of a diet rich in fruits and vegetables, including:

- decreased risk of developing type 2 diabetes
- lower blood pressure
- possible cancer-preventive effects
- reduced risk of cardiovascular disease, including heart attack and stroke

(Some of these studies also looked at the effects of eating whole grains, fiber, and nuts, in addition to fruits and vegetables.)

Based on current research, physicians recommend a diet rich in vegetables and fruits, our main sources of antioxidants.

Numerous clinical trials have investigated whether taking antioxidant supplements is helpful in preventing disease, but the results of those trials show no added benefits of taking antioxidant supplements. In fact, megadoses of vitamin E and beta-carotene may actually increase mortality. Remember, free radicals play some essential physiological roles, and removing all of them by consuming large doses of antioxidant supplements may actually increase the risk of certain chronic diseases.[1] Chapters 6 and 7 go into more detail about antioxidant supplements.

If you enjoy good underlying health, all you need is a healthy diet every day. Health benefits of a diet high in these plant foods are summarized in Figure 3.1.

lower risk of heart disease	lower risk of stroke	lower risk of various cancers	lower risk of type 2 diabetes	possible lower blood pressure

Figure 3.1. The advantages of eating a diet rich in fruits, vegetables, whole grains, and nuts

The Antioxidants Found in Fruits and Vegetables

A typical fruit and vegetable diet provides over 25,000 bioactive food constituents (also known as phytochemicals, because they are found in plants). Many phytochemicals are antioxidants, but the exact chemical nature and function of all the natural antioxidants are not fully understood even today.

In Chapter 1 we touched on the names of some of the antioxidants found in foods. This section goes into a bit more detail. Below are the major groups of antioxidants. This is not a comprehensive list.

Antioxidant Vitamins

Vitamins must be obtained from the diet because they are not manufactured by the body (with a couple of exceptions). There are three vitamins with specific antioxidant properties:

- **vitamin A (retinol)** — important for healthy skin, eyes, and immune function; found in animal products such as liver, egg yolks, whole milk, butter, and cheese
- **vitamin C (ascorbic acid)** — important in immune function, in wound healing, and for healthy teeth and gums; abundant in citrus fruits, strawberries, guava, mango, green vegetables, and peppers
- **vitamin E** — a complex mixture of eight compounds, of which alpha-tocopherol is the most common; excellent food sources include almonds, butternut squash, sunflower seeds, red bell peppers, and dark-green leafy vegetables

Carotenoids

Carotenoids are the main pigments responsible for the colors of fruits and vegetables. Chapter 1 lists three different types of carotenoids. In fact, there are over 600 different carotenoids, just a few of which are listed here:

- **astaxanthin** — another red pigment found in red- or pink-tinted seafood, as well as in red and orange fruits and vegetables such as carrots and red peppers

- **beta-carotene** — a precursor of vitamin A, and the most common carotenoid; top food sources include sweet potatoes, butternut squash, carrots, red bell peppers, spinach, kale, and pumpkin
- **beta-cryptoxanthin** — found in papaya, apples, egg yolks, and butter
- **lutein** — best known for its association with healthy eyes; abundant in green leafy vegetables such as collard greens, spinach, and kale; also found in egg yolks, animal fats, and the retina of the eyes
- **lycopene** — responsible for the red color of tomatoes and other fruits such as watermelon, papaya, pink grapefruit, apricot, and pink guava
- **zeaxanthin** — responsible for the red color of salmon; also found in trout, shrimp, krill, and crayfish

Polyphenols

Polyphenols, or phenolics, comprise a large category of phytochemicals that include flavonoids (the largest group), phenolic acids and esters, stilbenoids, and many others. The phenolics family is so large (over 8,000 different compounds have been identified) that it is difficult to generalize their possible health effects, but we know they are antioxidants. Most brightly colored fruits and vegetables supply polyphenols. Grapes, cherries, and berries are rich in these compounds. Caffeic acid, an antioxidant found in coffee, is part of the polyphenol family, as is resveratrol, found in grapes and red wine, and curcumin, found in turmeric.

Other Antioxidants

There are other important antioxidant compounds that are not carotenoids or polyphenolic compounds. One of these, capsaicin, found in chili peppers and chili powder, affords many health benefits.

Table 3.1 on the next page is for "chemistry geeks." It lists the chemical names of several of the major antioxidants (but not all of them). If you want to learn more about what these specific compounds do and what foods contain them, this table provides a starting point from which you can conduct your own research. However, knowing the names of all these chemicals is not necessary to understanding how antioxidants benefit your health and how to get plenty of them in your diet.

Which Foods Are Good Sources of Antioxidant Vitamins?

The rest of the chapter discusses the antioxidant content of various foods. Let's start with the antioxidant vitamins, C, A, and E. Unlike with other antioxidants, scientists working for the U.S. government have established suggested daily intakes — called recommended

TABLE 3.1. The Major Antioxidants

CLASS OF ANTIOXIDANT	INDIVIDUAL COMPOUND
Antioxidant Vitamins	Vitamin A, vitamin C, vitamin E
Carotenoids	Astaxanthin, beta-carotene, beta-cryptoxanthin, lutein, lycopene, zeaxanthin
Polyphenols	
Flavonoids	
Anthocyanins	Cyanidin, delphinidin, malvidin, pelargonidin, peonidin, and petunidin
Flavonols	Isorhamnetin, kaempferol, myricetin, quercetin
Flavan-3-ols	Catechins, epicatechin, epicatechin-3-gallate, epigallocatechin, gallocatechin, theaflavin, theaflavin-3-gallate, thearubigins
Flavones	Apigenin, luteolin
Flavanone	Eriodictyol, hesperetin, naringenin
Isoflavones	Daidzein, genistein
Phenolic Acids/Esters	cinnamic acid/derivatives, chlorogenic acid, gallic acid
Stilbenoids	Resveratrol
Other Phenolic Compounds	Curcumin
Other Antioxidants	Capsaicin

dietary allowances (RDAs) — for these nutrients, so it's relatively easy to figure out whether you're getting enough of them in your diet.

Vitamin C

Vegetables and fruits, especially citrus fruits, are important sources of vitamin C. Vitamin C, more than most other vitamins, is susceptible to breaking down when foods are cooked or improperly stored. For this reason, consuming fresh, raw fruits and vegetables maximizes the amount of vitamin C you can obtain from them. (This is not necessarily the case with all antioxidants, as you will see.) Moreover, it is better to store fruit whole rather than cut because vitamin C is more stable in whole fruit.

The vitamin C content of various fruits and vegetables is summarized in Table 3.2 on the next page. The RDA of vitamin C is 90 mg for men and 75 mg for women. (Smokers should add 35 mg to these recommendations.) The recommendations increase for women who are pregnant — to 85 mg — or breastfeeding — to 120 mg. You can see from the table that it is easy to obtain the recommended daily levels of vitamin C by eating one or two servings of certain fruits or vegetables.

Vitamin A/Beta-Carotene

Vitamin A, also called retinol, is found only in animal sources such as liver, egg yolks, and dairy fat. However, as mentioned, the pigment beta-carotene, found in many plant sources, is easily converted in the body into

TABLE 3.2. The Vitamin C Content of Various Fruits and Vegetables as per Common Measure (Source: USDA Website)

FOOD	WEIGHT (grams)	COMMON MEASURE	VITAMIN C (mg)
Asparagus, boiled	60	4 spears	14.6
Banana, raw	118	1 banana	10.3
Blackberries, raw	144	1 cup	30.2
Broccoli, raw	31	1 spear	27.7
Cabbage, raw	70	1 cup	27.6
Cauliflower, boiled	124	1 cup	54.9
Grapefruit juice, frozen	207	6-ounce can	248.0
Grapefruit, raw	118	½ grapefruit	39.3
Kiwi fruit, raw	76	1 medium fruit	70.5
Lime juice, raw	38	juice of 1 lime	11.4
Mango, raw	207	1 mango	75.3
Melon, cantaloupe, raw	160	1 cup	58.7
Melon, honeydew, raw	170	1 cup	30.6
Orange juice, frozen	213	6-ounce can	293.7
Orange juice, raw	248	1 cup	124.0
Orange, raw	131	1 orange	69.7
Papaya, raw	304	1 papaya	185.1
Peaches, frozen, sweetened	250	1 cup	235.5
Pepper, sweet, cooked	136	1 cup	190.3
Pineapple juice, canned, unsweetened	250	1 cup	25.0
Potato, boiled	156	1 cup	11.5
Raspberries, raw	123	1 cup	32.2
Spinach, raw	30	1 cup	8.4
Squash	205	1 cup	19.7
Strawberries, raw	166	1 cup	97.6
Tomatoes, red and ripe	240	1 cup	22.3

vitamin A. Two molecules of beta-carotene combine to form vitamin A, which is why the term "beta-carotene" is often used almost synonymously with "vitamin A."

The RDA of preformed vitamin A for adults is 900 micrograms (µg) for men and 700 µg for women per day. (You may also see vitamin A expressed in international units, IU, in which case the RDA is 3,000 IU and 2,310 IU, respectively.) During lactation, an additional 500–600 µg per day are recommended.

How much beta-carotene is recommended for good health? While there is currently no RDA for beta-carotene (like there is for vitamin A), U.S. government organizations such as the National Cancer Institute (NCI) and the Department of Agriculture (USDA) suggest a daily intake of about 6 mg. This amount is several times the average amount presently consumed in the United States (about 1.5 mg daily).

Table 3.3 on the next page lists the beta-carotene content of several fruits and vegetables. As with vitamin C, you can see that it is easy to reach or exceed your suggested daily intake of this important antioxidant by eating just a couple of servings of carefully selected fruits or vegetables.

Vitamin E

In addition to its activities as an antioxidant, vitamin E is involved in immune function, cell signaling, regulation of gene expression, and other metabolic processes. Vegetable oils (corn, olive, palm, safflower, soybean,

TABLE 3.3. The Beta-Carotene Content of Various Fruits and Vegetables as per Common Measure (Source: USDA Website)

FOOD	WEIGHT (grams)	COMMON MEASURE	BETA-CAROTENE (mg)
Broccoli, cooked	184	1 cup	1.1
Cabbage, raw	70	1 cup	4.7
Carrot juice, canned	236	1 cup	21.9
Carrots, raw	72	1 carrot	9.1
Green peas, cooked	160	1 cup	2.0
Lettuce, butterhead, raw	163	1 head	3.2
Lettuce, green leaf, raw	56	1 cup	2.9
Mango, raw	207	1 mango	1.3
Melon, cantaloupe, raw	160	1 cup	3.2
Okra, boiled	160	1 cup	2.7
Papaya, raw	304	1 papaya	8.3
Peaches, raw	170	1 cup	2.8
Pepper, sweet, red, raw	149	1 cup	2.4
Pumpkin, canned, no salt	245	1 cup	17.0
Pumpkin, cooked	245	1 cup	5.1
Spinach, boiled	180	1 cup	11.3
Sweet potato, cooked	156	1 potato	16.8
Tomato, red, ripe, raw	180	1 cup	7.7
Watermelon, raw	286	1 wedge	8.7
Winter squash, cooked	205	1 cup	5.7

sunflower, etc.), nuts, wheat germ, and whole grains are the most important sources of vitamin E. Other sources include seeds, certain fish, and green leafy vegetables. The RDA for vitamin E for healthy adult men and women is 15 mg (22.4 IU). For women who are breast-feeding it's 19 mg (28.3 IU). To convert milligrams of vitamin E to IU, multiply the number of milligrams by 1.49.

Table 3.4 on the next page lists the vitamin E content of various foods. Although the focus of this chapter is primarily on fruits and vegetables, other foods are included in this table. That's because, with a few exceptions, fruits and vegetables aren't the best sources of vitamin E.

The Antioxidant Rankings of Various Foods and the Effects of Cooking

Now let's approach the issue of antioxidant content in foods from a different angle. Many experiments show that an intake of foods rich in the antioxidant vitamins (C, A, and E) is associated with a decrease in diseases related to oxidative stress. However, as mentioned above, large studies testing the effectiveness of supplements of these vitamins don't seem to show the same benefits. As researcher B. L. Halvorsen states:

> One possible explanation may be that the bene-ficial health effect is contributed by other anti-oxidants in fruit and vegetables.... We suggest

TABLE 3.4. The Vitamin E Content of Various Foods as per Common Measure (Source: USDA Website)

FOOD	WEIGHT (gm)	COMMON MEASURE	VITAMIN E (mg)
Blackberries, raw	144	1 cup	1.7
Blueberries, raw	145	1 cup	0.83
Broccoli, chopped, cooked	184	1 cup	2.4
Carrot juice, canned	236	1 cup	2.7
Fish, rainbow trout	85	3 ounces	2.4
Fish, salmon, cooked	85	3 ounces	1.0
Fish, swordfish	106	1 piece	2.6
Kiwi fruit, raw	76	1 medium	1.1
Mango, raw	207	1 mango	1.9
Nuts, almonds	28.3	24 nuts	7.4
Oil, canola	14	1 tablespoon	2.4
Oil, corn	13.6	1 tablespoon	1.9
Oil, olive	13.6	1 tablespoon	1.9
Papaya, raw	304	1 papaya	0.9
Pinto beans, cooked	171	1 cup	1.6
Peaches, raw	170	1 cup	1.2
Peanuts, dry roasted with salt	28.35	28 peanuts	2.1
Peppers, raw, sweet, red	119	1 pepper	1.9
Raspberries, raw	123	1 cup	1.1
Spinach, frozen, chopped, cooked	190	1 cup	6.7
Sunflower oil	13.6	1 tablespoon	5.6

that these redox-active compounds [i.e., antioxidants], which cooperate in an integrated manner in plant cells, also may cooperate in animal cells. Thus, a network of antioxidants with different chemical properties may be needed for proper protection against oxidative damage.[2]

In other words, you have to eat a varied diet filled with antioxidant-rich foods, not just take megadoses of supplements. (See Chapters 6 and 7 for more on this topic.)

Halvorsen and colleagues published an excellent paper in 2006 ranking certain foods by their antioxidant content. The top thirty foods are listed in Table 3.5 on the next page.

To determine a food's antioxidant content, these scientists used a test called the FRAP test, which is different from the ORAC test. (FRAP stands for ferric-reducing ability of plasma.)

The same authors also studied the effects of cooking on the antioxidant content of food. Interestingly, for some foods the antioxidant content *increases* during cooking, because antioxidant compounds become more available due to the breakdown of cells. Although older publications promoted consuming raw vegetables whenever possible, more recent studies suggest that cooking often increases the availability of antioxidants in vegetables. The effects of cooking on certain foods' antioxidant capacity are summarized in Table 3.6 on page 41.

TABLE 3.5. The Foods with the Highest Antioxidant Content per Serving

RANK	FOOD
1	Blackberries
2	Walnuts
3	Strawberries
4	Antichokes, prepared
5	Cranberries
6	Coffee
7	Raspberries
8	Pecans
9	Blueberries
10	Cloves, ground
11	Grape juice
12	Chocolate, baked, unsweetened
13	Cherries, sour
14	Power Bar, chocolate flavor
15	Guava nectar
16	Juice drinks (10% juice, blueberry or strawberry, vitamin C)
17	Cranapple juice
18	Prunes
19	Chocolate, dark, sugar free
20	Cabbage, red, cooked
21	Orange juice
22	Apple juice with vitamin C
23	Mango nectar
24	Pineapple
25	Oranges
26	Bran Flakes breakfast cereal (Ralston Food)
27	Plums, black
28	Pinto beans, dried
29	Canned chili with meat, no beans
30	Spinach, frozen

TABLE 3.6. The Effects of Cooking on Selected Foods

FOOD	TYPE OF COOKING	ANTIOXIDANT CONTENT AS PERCENT OF UNCOOKED FOOD

FOOD WITH INCREASED ANTIOXIDANT CONTENT AFTER COOKING

FOOD	TYPE OF COOKING	ANTIOXIDANT CONTENT AS PERCENT OF UNCOOKED FOOD
Asparagus	Cooking by steaming	205%
Bagels	Toasting	134–367%
Broccoli	Cooking by steaming	122–654%
Cabbage	Cooking by steaming	448%
Carrots	Boiling	121–159%
Carrots	Cooking by steaming	291%
Carrots	Microwave cooking	113–143%
Green peppers	Cooking by steaming	467%
Mushrooms	Microwave cooking	113%
Pie crust	Baking	311–1450%
Potatoes	Cooking by steaming	105–242%
Red cabbage	Cooking by steaming	270%
Red pepper	Cooking by steaming	180%
Spinach	Boiling	84–114%
Spinach	Microwave cooking	103–121%
Sweet potatoes	Boiling	413%
Tomatoes	Cooking by steaming	112–164%
Wheat bread	Toasting	153–185%

FOODS WITH DECREASED ANTIOXIDANT CONTENT AFTER COOKING

FOOD	TYPE OF COOKING	ANTIOXIDANT CONTENT AS PERCENT OF UNCOOKED FOOD
Corn grits	Microwave cooking	21–32%
Spaghetti	Cooking by steaming	42–63%
White rice	Cooking by steaming	33–70%

Cooking may increase antioxidant capacity of some vegetables by making antioxidant compounds more readily available for absorption by the gut.

The Recommended Intake of Antioxidants

If you remember from Chapter 1, one of the most common methods of measuring antioxidant levels in foods is what is known as the ORAC score. In general, although there is no RDA established for antioxidants, it has been suggested that a total daily intake of an ORAC value of around 5,000 is a good goal. A daily ORAC value of 7,000 may be even more desirable. A target ORAC value of 5,000 can be easily achieved by eating enough fruits and vegetables every day. Remember the proverb "An apple a day keeps the doctor away"? It may be more than just an old saying. Eating just one average-size Golden Delicious apple will provide you with an approximate ORAC value of 4,005.

If you get even five servings of your favorite fruits and vegetables per day you will easily reach an ORAC value of 7,000. A great strategy is to eat the fruits and vegetables you enjoy, but I will suggest that making it a point every day to eat a serving of any berry that you like (e.g., strawberries, blueberries, raspberries) and a serving of any nut that you like (e.g., almonds, hazelnuts, walnuts) is the best way to reach a high ORAC value. You could even try keeping doctors away with açai fruit, which is very high on the antioxidant list.

The rest of the chapter summarizes the ORAC values of many fruits, vegetables, and other foods. The values listed are expressed as *micromole Trolox equivalent (TE) per 100 grams* (µTE/100 g). For folks who aren't scientists, what's important about that number is the "per 100 grams" part.

When you encounter a huge number like 290,283 µTE (the ORAC score for ground cloves), you must remember that it refers to the ORAC value contained in 100 grams of ground cloves, *not in a typical serving of cloves*. A normal serving of cloves might be more like 0.5 grams — which equals about ¼ teaspoon — or even less. Thus, a single serving (¼ teaspoon) of ground cloves has an ORAC value of about 1,451, still quite high. (You will notice that several spices and herbs have high ORAC scores.)

On the other hand, when we're talking about fruits and vegetables, 100 grams is close to a normal serving size. A hundred grams roughly equals 3.5 ounces, which is about ⅔ cup of blueberries, or about 1 cup of chopped broccoli. An average-size apple is about 150 grams. The point here is to think about what a reasonable serving size is. A good resource to help you compare quantity in grams to normal serving sizes is www.fatsecret.com /calories-nutrition.

> It's important to be aware of serving sizes when researching the ORAC value of a food. Although ORAC scores are usually expressed per 100 grams of a food, not all foods are eaten in 100 gram portions. Spices, for example, are typically consumed in much smaller portions.

A part of the controversy surrounding ORAC values is due to the fact that it's easy for people to be confused by the portion size. Pay attention to this detail when thinking about the ORAC scores of foods you eat.

The ORAC values in this chapter originally came from the USDA website. As discussed in Chapter 1, the USDA no longer publishes ORAC ratings on its website. However, as of this book's publication date, other websites continue to post ORAC scores, including www.oracvalues.com. (The ORAC numbers presented here may not match numbers presented by other resources because some investigators express ORAC values in other units.)

The Fruits Rich in Antioxidants

Among the fruits commonly consumed in the United States, certain berries have the highest antioxidant capacity, probably because of their high levels of anthocyanins, water-soluble pigments found mostly in the skin of berry fruits.

> Berries are probably the best antioxidant fruits
> available.

All berries are great sources of antioxidants, but chokeberry and cranberry have particularly high antioxidant activity. Blueberries, blackberries, raspberries, and strawberries are also excellent dietary sources of antioxidants. Table 3.7 lists the ORAC values of some common berries.

TABLE 3.7. The ORAC Scores of Various Berry Fruits

BERRY FRUIT	ORAC VALUE (µTE/100 g)
Blackberry	5,905
Blueberry	4,669
Chokeberry	16,062
Cranberry	9,090
Raspberry	5,065
Strawberry	4,302

Table 3.8 on the next page lists the ORAC values for other common fruits. You will notice that cherries rank high on the list. Cherries, especially sweet cherries, are dense with nutrients, including antioxidants. These bioactive components of cherries are responsible for reduction in the risk of cardiovascular disease, diabetes, inflammatory diseases, and Alzheimer's disease.[3] Another fruit high on the list is the açai berry, the fruit

of the açai palm, which is traditionally consumed in Brazil and is becoming popular in other countries because of its high antioxidant content. In one study, the antioxidant capacity of the blood was increased two- to threefold after consumption of açai juice and palms by volunteers.[4] Dried fruits have higher ORAC scores (per 100 grams) than their fresh counterparts, of course, because everything — from sugar to antioxidants — is more concentrated in a dehydrated fruit. Finally, note that for most fruits (e.g., apples) it is important to eat the skin to obtain the greatest antioxidant benefit. That's because many antioxidants are actually pigments, which are located primarily in a fruit's skin.

TABLE 3.8. The ORAC Scores of Common Fruits and Fruit Juices

FRUIT/FRUIT JUICE	ORAC VALUE (µTE/100 g)
Açai fruit, pulp/skin	102,700
Apple, Fuji, raw with skin	2,589
Apple, Golden Delicious, raw with skin	2,670
Apple, Red Delicious, raw with skin	2,936
Apricots, raw	1,110
Avocado	1,922
Banana, raw	795
Cantaloupe, raw	319
Cherries, sweet, raw	3,747
Dates	3,895
Grapefruit, raw, pink	1,640
Grapes, green	1,018
Grapes, black	1,746

(cont'd.)

TABLE 3.8. The ORAC Scores of Common Fruits and Fruit Juices (cont'd.)

FRUIT/FRUIT JUICE	ORAC VALUE (µTE/100 g)
Guava, common, raw	1,422
Kiwi fruit, fresh, raw	862
Lemon, raw	1,346
Lime, raw	82
Mango, raw	1,300
Melon, honeydew, raw	253
Nectarine, raw	919
Orange, raw	2,103
Papaya, raw	300
Peach, raw	1,922
Pear, raw	1,746
Pineapple, raw	562
Plum, dried (prune), uncooked	8,059
Plum, raw	6,100
Pomegranate, raw	4,479
Raisins, golden seedless	10,450
Tangerine (Mandarin orange)	1,627
Watermelon	142

COMMON FRUIT JUICES

Apple juice (canned or bottled, unsweetened)	414
Cranberry juice (unsweetened)	1,452
Grapefruit juice, white	1,238
Grape juice, concord	2,389
Grape juice, white	793
Lemon juice	1,225
Orange juice, canned, unsweetened	703
Orange juice, raw	726

The Vegetables Rich in Antioxidants

Like fruits, many vegetables are good sources of antioxidants. Dark green vegetables such as broccoli, leafy lettuces, kale, and spinach are all rich in antioxidants.

Researchers in one study concluded that consumption of dark yellow and orange vegetables was consistently more predictive of reduced risk of cancer in a certain sample of the population than any other food group.[5] Sweet potatoes are rich in antioxidant compounds, including phenolic compounds, vitamin C, and carotenoids. In general the antioxidant capacity of sweet potatoes is increased after cooking.[6] Among other vegetables, artichokes, asparagus, beets, and red cabbage are good sources of antioxidants.

The ORAC values of various vegetables are summarized in Table 3.9.

TABLE 3.9. The ORAC Scores of Common Vegetables

VEGETABLES	ORAC VALUE (µTE/100 g)
BEANS AND PEAS	
Black beans, raw	8,494
Black beans, boiled	2,249
Garbanzo beans (chickpeas)	847
Green beans, raw	799
Kidney beans	8,606
Lentils	7,282
Navy beans, raw	8,320
Pinto beans, raw	8,033
Pinto beans, boiled	904

(cont'd.)

Research indicates that dark-green, red, and orange vegetables are high in carotenoids, including beta-carotene, lycopene, and lutein, which are excellent antioxidants. In addition, oxygenated carotenoids known as xanthophylls are also found in these vegetables.

TABLE 3.9. The ORAC Scores of Common Vegetables (cont'd.)

VEGETABLES	ORAC VALUE (µTE/100 g)
Soy beans, raw	962
Split peas	524
DARK GREEN VEGETABLES	
Broccoli, boiled	2,160
Broccoli, raw	1,510
Dark green leafy lettuce, raw	1,532
Kale	1,770
Romaine lettuce, raw	1,017
Spinach, raw	1,513
RED AND ORANGE VEGETABLES	
Butternut squash	396
Carrots, boiled	326
Carrots, raw	697
Pumpkin, raw	483
Red peppers, sweet, raw	821
Sweet potatoes, baked in skin	2,115
Sweet potatoes, cooked, boiled without skin	766
Sweet potatoes, raw	902
Tomatoes, red, ripe, cooked	423
Tomatoes, red, ripe, raw	387

(cont'd.)

TABLE 3.9. The ORAC Scores of Common Vegetables (cont'd.)

VEGETABLES	ORAC VALUE (µTE/100 g)
STARCHY VEGETABLES	
Corn, sweet, yellow, raw	728
Green peas	600
Lima beans	243
Potatoes, red, raw	1,098
Potatoes, white, flesh and skin baked	1,138
Potatoes, red, flesh and skin baked	1,326
OTHER VEGETABLES	
Artichokes, boiled	9,416
Artichokes, microwaved	9,402
Artichokes, raw	6,552
Asparagus, cooked, boiled, drained	1,644
Asparagus, raw	2,252
Beets, raw	1,776
Brussels sprouts	980
Cabbage, boiled	856
Cabbage, raw	529
Cabbage, red, boiled	3,145
Cabbage, red, raw	2,496
Cauliflower, raw	833
Celery	552
Cucumbers, raw	140
Eggplant, boiled	245
Eggplant, raw	932
Green peppers	935
Iceberg (head) lettuce	438
Mushrooms, portobello	968
Mushrooms, shiitake	752

(cont'd.)

TABLE 3.9. The ORAC Scores of Common Vegetables (cont'd.)

VEGETABLES	ORAC VALUE (μTE/100 g)
Onions, red, raw	1,521
Onions, white, raw	863
Onions, yellow, sautéed	1,220
Parsley, raw	1,301
Yellow squash	150
Zucchini	180

The Spices and Herbs Rich in Antioxidants

Spices are the richest source of antioxidants. Research indicates that although spices are minor dietary constituents, they have antioxidant, antimicrobial, and anticancer properties and are good for health.[7] Cinnamon has antioxidant, anti-inflammatory, antitumor, and antibacterial activity. In addition, cinnamon may be useful in lowering cholesterol and controlling blood sugar because it acts as an insulin mimetic.[8] Other researchers have described the potential health benefits of Indian spices in treating various symptoms such as hypertension, diabetes, and obesity.[9] Herbs, which are seasonings that come from the leafy parts of plants (e.g., basil, oregano), can be thought of as leafy green vegetables that are consumed in tiny portions.

Again, with spices and herbs, although the ORAC values listed in Table 3.10 on the next page are expressed in units per 100 grams, remember that you will most likely eat a much smaller serving size than that — often less than a single gram at any one time.

TABLE 3.10. The ORAC Values of Common Spices, Herbs, and Other Seasonings

SPICE/HERB/SEASONING	ORAC VALUE (µTE/100 g)
Basil, dried	61,063
Basil, fresh	4,805
Cardamom	2,764
Chili powder	23,636
Cinnamon, ground	131,420
Cloves, ground	290,283
Cumin seed	50,372
Curry powder	48,504
Garlic powder	6,665
Ginger, dried, ground	39,041
Mustard seed, yellow	29,257
Nutmeg	69,640
Oregano, dried	175,295
Oregano, fresh	13,970
Peppermint, fresh	13,987
Paprika	21,932
Parsley, dried	73,670
Red pepper (cayenne)	19,671
Rosemary	165,280
Sage, ground	119,929
Thyme, dried	157,380
Turmeric, ground	127,068
Vanilla bean	122,400
Vinegar, apple and honey	270
Vinegar, honey	225
Vinegar, red wine	410

The Nuts Rich in Antioxidants

Nuts are excellent sources of antioxidants. Peanuts, although they are legumes rather than nuts, are also rich in antioxidants. Consuming nuts and peanut butter even once a week can reduce the risk of coronary heart disease. In one study, the highest risk reduction was observed in subjects who consumed nuts or peanut butter one to four times a week.[10] Epidemiological studies clearly indicate that regular consumption of nuts and peanuts can reduce the incidence of sudden death from heart disease. Nuts and peanuts can decrease the concentration of cholesterol in the blood.[11] The antioxidant compounds in nuts can improve lipid profiles, reduce risk of heart diseases, and improve health without weight gain.[12]

The ORAC values of various nuts are summarized in Table 3.11 on the next page. A reasonable serving size of nuts is about 1 ounce (approximately ¼ cup for most nuts). By contrast, 100 grams (the unit expressed here) equals 3.5 ounces, quite a bit larger than a typical serving size for nuts.

Organic vs. Conventional?

When it comes to antioxidant levels in organic versus conventionally grown produce, researchers have reported different results on this question. Let's look at several recent scientific articles.

One study showed that organically grown sweet bell pepper had higher levels of antioxidants such as

TABLE 3.11. The ORAC Scores of Common Nuts

NUT	ORAC VALUE (µTE/100 g)
Almonds	4,454
Cashews	1,948
Hazelnuts	9,645
Macadamia nuts	1,695
Peanuts (technically a legume)	3,166
Pecans	17,940
Pistachios	7,675
Walnuts	13,541

carotenoids, phenolic compounds, and vitamin C compared to conventionally grown sweet peppers.[13] Tomatoes grown organically were found to have more vitamin C and antioxidants.[14] The micronutrient content (vitamins, minerals, and other phytochemicals) was more commonly higher in organically grown vegetables and legumes compared to their conventional counterparts.[15] Organically grown eggplant had higher potassium, calcium, magnesium, and antioxidants (total phenolic compounds) than eggplant grown under conventional conditions.[16]

However, in another article, the authors found no difference between the content of bioactive compounds in tomatoes grown under organic conditions versus conventional conditions.[17]

There may be other compelling reasons to eat organic foods — for example, wanting to avoid consuming pesticide residues — but in terms of antioxidant content the research is inconclusive on the merits of organic versus conventional produce.

The Antioxidants in Other Foods

In addition to eating fruits and vegetables each day we need to get enough carbohydrates and proteins in our diet. Fortified breakfast cereals may be a good source of antioxidants and dietary fibers. Typically, the ORAC values of fortified breakfast cereals vary between 1,000 and 2,500 per 100 grams of cereal (a normal serving size is anywhere between 20 and 50 grams). By contrast, bread, rice, pasta, and other grain foods are not rich in antioxidants.

Meat and fish are relatively poor sources of most antioxidants, although they are high in protein and beneficial for health in other ways. Eating fish or taking fish oil supplements offers health benefits including a lower risk of cardiovascular disease.

It is very clear that we need to eat fruits and vegetables every day, not only to get enough antioxidants but also because they contain vitamins, minerals, and other beneficial nutrients. Consuming at least five servings of fruits and vegetables should be considered the bare minimum; nine or ten servings a day is a good practice. Eating out is fun, but try to avoid fast food — instead, stick to full-service restaurants where you can order vegetable dishes.

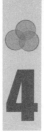

The Antioxidants in Tea, Coffee, and Chocolate

4

Caffeine is the most widely consumed psychoactive compound in the world. A majority of adults consume it on a daily basis, most commonly through drinking coffee or tea. Fortunately, both beverages are rich in antioxidants that provide many health benefits. Chocolate, too, is a rich source of antioxidants, but it is high in calories. Tea, coffee, and chocolate in the right amounts can be healthy foods for people (but do not allow your pet cat or dog to consume any of these substances, because they contain theobromine, which may be fatal to animals if too much is consumed).

The Antioxidants in Tea and Coffee

Both coffee and tea are rich in antioxidants, but the antioxidant capacity of human blood is increased more after drinking coffee because coffee is endowed with an antioxidant content five to eight times greater than that of tea.

Contrary to popular belief, a cup of coffee provides more antioxidants than a cup of tea.

The major antioxidants found in both tea and coffee are broadly called polyphenolic compounds, which are substances the plant produces to help defend itself against diseases caused by microorganisms such as bacteria or fungi. (See Chapter 3 for more about polyphenolic compounds.) In addition, green tea contains a subcategory of polyphenols called catechins, which are usually not found in coffee. Because black tea is produced by fermentation, the catechins in it have undergone a chemical transformation to form the antioxidant compound thearubigin.

Caffeic acid and its derivative chlorogenic acid are the major sources of antioxidants in coffee. Coffee also contains many minor components with significant antioxidant capacity. One group of researchers estimated the amount of antioxidants in a cup of coffee, combined that data with the U.S per capita consumption of coffee (estimated at 1.9 cups per day for men and 1.4 cups for women), and concluded that coffee is probably the number-one source of antioxidants in the American diet.[1]

For overall health, it is generally better to drink filtered coffee rather than boiled coffee or espresso because of two other components of coffee: cafestol and kahweol, which can increase cholesterol levels. These chemicals are trapped by coffee filter paper, so an almost negligible amount is found in filtered coffee.

The various components of tea and coffee, as well as their ORAC values, are summarized in Table 4.1 below.

Note the high ORAC value of 100 grams of coffee compared to the same quantity of tea. (Again, while some readers may find these chemical names interesting, it is not necessary to be familiar with them in order to reap their benefits.)

TABLE 4.1. The Components and ORAC Scores of Tea and Coffee

BEVERAGE	COMPONENTS	ORAC VALUE (μTE/100 g)
Black tea	**Antioxidants:** theaflavins, thearubigins, smaller amounts of catechins than green tea **Other Components:** amino acids, caffeine, theobromine, theophylline	1,153
Green tea	**Antioxidants:** epicatechin, epicatechin gallate, epigallocatechin, epigallocatechin gallate, kaempferol, myristicin, quercetin **Other Components:** amino acids, caffeine, theobromine, theophylline	1,253
Coffee	**Antioxidants:** caffeic acid, chlorogenic acid, dihydro-caffeic acid **Other Components:** cafestol, caffeine, theobromine, kahweol	up to 15,264 (depending on the type of coffee bean)

The Health Benefits of Tea

In general, three types of tea are consumed worldwide, but all are produced from the young leaves of the same plant: *Camellia sinensis*. Depending on the processing, tea can be subdivided into black tea, green tea, and oolong tea. Green tea is favored in most parts of China, in Japan, and in certain other Asian countries. Black tea is favored in Western countries and the Indian sub-continent. Oolong is favored by the people of southern China.

Green tea is produced in Japan by steaming tea leaves and in China by panning (pan-frying). These processes destroy enzymes, preventing further biotransformation of tea components. Green tea retains the original color of the tea leaves. Black tea is produced by full fermenta-tion (oxidation) of tea leaves. Oolong tea is partially fer-mented, which lends it an excellent character, combin-ing the aroma of black tea and the freshness of green tea.

The increased antioxidant capacity of the blood after drinking either black or green tea has been well docu-mented in the medical literature. Drinking tea regularly can decrease oxidative stress in the body, perhaps help-ing to prevent cancer and reducing occurrence of heart diseases.[2] The total antioxidant capacity of human blood after drinking either black or green tea is increased by a similar magnitude, although some investigators claim that green tea has better antioxidant potential than black tea.[3] However, as you can see from Table 4.1 on the previous page, the ORAC values of brewed green tea and brewed black tea are similar (1,253 versus 1,153).

The potential health benefits of drinking tea (both black and green) are as follows:

- anti-inflammatory effects
- boosting immune system
- enhanced mental alertness

- less chance of cognitive impairment due to dementia
- possible antidepressant properties
- possible increase in bone health (green tea)
- possible prevention of various types of cancer
- possible reduction in blood cholesterol levels
- possible reduction in blood pressure
- possible reduction in obesity (green tea)
- reduced levels of cortisol, the primary stress hormone (green tea)
- reduced risk of heart disease, including heart attack
- reduced risk of stroke

The Health Benefits of Coffee

Coffee is a brewed beverage made from the roasted beans (seeds) of the *Coffea* plant. The beans are found in coffee berries or "cherries." Coffee bushes are grown in many countries, primarily at latitudes close to the equator. Coffee is sometimes served as espresso, which is simply a different way of brewing coffee, resulting in a much stronger extraction.

Coffee contains more caffeine than tea, depending, of course, on the strength of the brew. An average cup of coffee contains 181 mg of caffeine, versus an average of 130 mg in a cup of tea. Excessive caffeine intake can cause insomnia and restlessness, and can increase blood pressure by stimulation of the central nervous system, but such effects are typically not observed if a person drinks four or fewer cups of coffee per day. Furthermore, caffeine intake greater than 250 mg per day may cause caffeine dependence.

Of course, one way to keep caffeine intake low is to drink decaffeinated coffee, which contains a very small amount of caffeine (approximately 3 mg per cup). Despite the downsides of excessive caffeine intake, drinking coffee in moderation offers many beneficial health effects because of its high antioxidant content. And consuming small amounts of caffeine can afford some advantages, too.

Drinking one or two cups a day of regular coffee can improve mental alertness and cognitive function, mostly due to caffeine.

The potential health benefits of drinking coffee are as follows:

- improved alertness and cognitive function
- laxative effect
- prevention of gallstones and diseases of the gall-bladder
- reduced risk of cirrhosis of the liver
- reduced risk of coronary heart disease
- reduced risk of depression
- reduced risk of gout

- reduced risk of Parkinson's disease
- reduced risk of suicide
- reduced risk of type 2 diabetes
- reduced risk of various types of cancers (breast, colon, kidney, liver)

However, drinking coffee isn't all beneficial. Drinking excessive amounts of coffee may prevent the body from absorbing iron and other minerals. Women who want to get pregnant or who are pregnant should avoid drinking too much coffee. Studies indicate that women who consume 400–800 mg of caffeine (more than two cups of coffee) each day may experience significant delays in getting pregnant. Some experts maintain that an intake of caffeine greater than 300 mg a day (one and a half cups of coffee) may increase the risk of spontaneous abortion, although this finding has been disputed. No study has ever linked birth defects with consumption of coffee in pregnant women.[4]

How Much Tea or Coffee?

In general, drinking three to five cups of tea per day (green tea or a combination of green and black tea) is sufficient to reap tea's health benefits. If you drink more than five cups of tea a day, it probably won't cause any harm.

If you drink regular coffee, limit your intake to two or three eight-ounce cups, to avoid the possible detrimental side effects of too much caffeine. A daily caffeine intake of 300 to 400 mg a day (up to three cups) may not cause any harm unless the person has a genetic problem metabolizing caffeine. If you have unstable blood pressure you probably should stick to decaffeinated coffee. A woman who is pregnant or who wants to get pregnant should not drink more than one cup of regular coffee per day, and may want to consider drinking only decaffeinated coffee.

Coffee and tea by themselves contain almost no calories, but adding milk and sugar can increase the caloric value to approximately 50 calories per serving. Moreover, some of the sugary coffee drinks available at most gourmet coffee shops can contain as many as 400 calories!

If you like both beverages, experts currently recommend up to 40 ounces (five cups total) per day of tea, coffee, or a combination of the two.

The Antioxidants in Chocolate

The cacao tree (*Theobroma cacao*) was probably first cultivated in 250–900 AD by the people of the ancient Mayan civilization in Mexico and Central America. Following the Spanish conquest of Mexico, cocoa beans were introduced to Spain in 1528. Over the next century, Europeans learned to add various substances to cocoa such as sugar, vanilla, and cinnamon to mask its naturally bitter taste. Chocolate was introduced to North America around the mid-1800s. It is now a favorite food product throughout the world.

The seeds or beans of the cacao tree must be fermented, dried, or roasted in order to prepare chocolate. Much of the chocolate consumed today is sweet chocolate, combining cocoa solids, cocoa butter or another fat, and sugar. Milk chocolate also contains milk powder or condensed milk. White chocolate contains cocoa butter, sugar, and milk, but no cocoa solids.

Chocolate has excellent antioxidant properties. The primary antioxidants present in chocolate are catechin, epicatechin, and proanthocyanidins. Dark chocolate is formulated with a higher percentage of cocoa bean liquor and therefore contains more antioxidants than milk chocolate. Dry cocoa powder (unsweetened) also contains high amounts of antioxidants. The ORAC values of various forms of chocolate are listed in Table 4.2. One hundred grams of chocolate (about 3.5 ounces) is roughly equivalent to two good-sized chocolate bars.

TABLE 4.2. The ORAC Values of Chocolate

TYPE OF CHOCOLATE	ORAC VALUE (µTE/100 g)
Baking chocolate, unsweetened	49,093
Chocolate syrup	6,330
Cocoa, dry powder, unsweetened	55,653
Dark chocolate	20,816
Milk chocolate	7,519
Semi-sweet chocolate	18,053

The Health Benefits (and Drawbacks) of Chocolate

Currently, it has been accepted that the major health benefit of eating chocolate is a lower risk of heart diseases, including heart attack. Unfortunately, as we all know, chocolate is full of calories. A hundred grams of chocolate may contain 400–500 calories, or even more. A significant amount of fat is naturally present in cocoa butter. Currently, consumption of no more than 25 grams (about one ounce) per day of dark chocolate is recommended for the prevention of heart diseases and to gain the other health benefits of dark chocolate. Although it is tempting to do so, avoid eating chocolate with milk because milk proteins may inhibit absorption of the beneficial antioxidant flavonoids contained in chocolate. This is also why milk chocolate affords fewer health benefits than dark chocolate.

Eating dark chocolate is better than eating milk chocolate because dark chocolate contains fewer calories and contains higher amounts of antioxidants.

The potential benefits of eating chocolate are:
- better blood-sugar control in diabetics
- improved flow of blood through arteries
- lower blood pressure
- may lower triglycerides

- lower risk of various cardiovascular diseases, including heart attack
- may improve concentration of "good" cholesterol (HDL)
- thinner blood

The primary drawback to eating too much chocolate is the consumption of excess calories, leading to possible weight gain. Diabetics also need to pay attention to the sugar content of chocolate.

The Antioxidants in Red Wine and Other Alcoholic Beverages

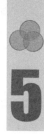

5

The origins of consuming alcohol may be traceable back to our ape ancestors forty million years ago. Yeasts that naturally occur in fruit convert sugars into ethanol (alcohol). An "alcoholic" smell indicates that the fruit is ripe and ready to eat. In tropical forests, hungry primates capable of identifying ripe foods by their particular odor survived better than others, and eventually "natural selection" favored apes with a keen appreciation for the smell and taste of alcohol. It is possible that the human taste for alcohol arose during our long-shared ancestry with primates.[1]

Alcoholic beverages can be classified into three broad categories: beer, wine, and spirits. Beer and wine are fermented beverages. Hard liquors or spirits are produced using fermentation followed by distillation. The alcohol content of different alcoholic beverages varies widely due to variability in serving size, but a standard drink contains approximately 14 grams of alcohol. Alcoholic drinks consist of water, alcohol, variable amounts of sugars, and carbohydrates (residual sugar and starch left after fermentation). Distilled alcoholic beverages such as spirits are devoid of any residual sugar. Usually one standard drink contains 100–140 calories.

Moderate Drinking Versus Hazardous Drinking

Alcohol is a double-edged sword. Drinking it in moderate amounts can offer many beneficial effects, but heavy drinking is very hazardous to human health. Guidelines for moderate alcohol consumption, provided by the U.S. government, are as follows:[2]

Men: No more than two standard alcoholic drinks per day; 14 drinks per week

Women: No more than one standard alcoholic drink per day; 7 drinks per week

Adults over sixty-five (both male and female): No more than 1 drink per day

A standard serving of alcohol is considered to be 5 fluid ounces of wine, 12 fluid ounces of beer, or 1.5 fluid ounces of spirits.

Consuming five or more drinks in one day may be harmful, even if a person does so only once a month. A London-based study of over 10,000 government employees between ages 35 and 55 with an eleven-year follow-up concluded that optimal drinking is once or twice per week with a daily consumption of one drink or less. People who consumed alcohol even twice a day had an increased risk of mortality from various causes (diseases) compared to those drinking once or twice a week.[3]

An additional consideration is the caloric content of alcohol beverages. Drinking too many calories can lead to weight gain. In addition, diabetics should pay attention to the sugar content of beer, wine, and some cocktails.

Finally, although the antioxidant effects of moderate alcohol intake are fairly well documented, if consumed in excess, alcohol can act as a pro-oxidant, meaning it *promotes* oxidative stress in the body. Heavy drinking both increases oxidative stress *and* depletes nutrients responsible for protecting the body from oxidative stress.

The Health Benefits of Moderate Drinking

The health benefits of drinking in moderation are summarized in Table 5.1 on the next page. In general, wine, especially red wine, is superior to other alcoholic beverages due to its high antioxidant content. Pregnant women should abstain from all drinking to avoid miscarriage, stillbirth, and birth of a child with fetal alcohol syndrome.

In particular, quite a few studies have found that drinking in moderation reduces the risk of heart disease and heart attack. Several theories, summarized below, have been proposed about why this may be true.

Moderate alcohol consumption:
- increases the concentration of "good" cholesterol (HDL cholesterol)
- increases coronary blood flow

TABLE 5.1. The Benefits of Drinking in Moderation

BENEFITS	COMMENTS
Increased longevity	Antioxidants have an antiaging effect.
Reduced chance of catching the common cold	Red wine helps protect against colds. (Beer and spirits had no effect, in one study.)
Reduced risk of certain types of cancers	Beer and wine may protect against some cancers.
Reduced risk of dementia/Alzheimer's	Red wine is superior to other alcoholic beverages for protection due to the presence of the antioxidant resveratrol.
Reduced risk of developing arthritis	Alcohol provides some protection.
Reduced risk of forming gallstones	Alcohol provides some protection.
Reduced risk of heart disease	One drink or less per day can protect the heart. Red wine may provide more protection than white wine due to the presence of higher amounts of polyphenolic antioxidants.
Reduced risk of stroke	Moderate drinking is the key, and again red wine is superior.

- decreases the concentration of "bad" cholesterol (LDL cholesterol)
- reduces the narrowing of coronary arteries by reducing plaque formation
- reduces the risk of blood clotting
- reduces the level of fibrinogen, a blood-clotting factor
- reduces blood pressure, especially in females

Red Wine: Superior to Other Alcoholic Beverages

Wine, especially red wine, produces more health benefits than beer because wine provides more antioxidants. Red wine is made from the must (pulp) of red or black grapes, crushed with the grape skins. By contrast, white wine is usually made by fermenting the juice pressed from white grapes (or, in the case of rosé, from red grapes) with very little or no grape skin. Grape skin is full of antioxidants. Scientists have demonstrated that these compounds are found in more abundance in red wine compared to white wine.[4] See Table 5.2. The point of this table isn't for you to memorize the names and amounts of antioxidant compounds found in red versus white wine, but rather to have a point of comparison between the two.

TABLE 5.2. The Major Antioxidant Compounds Found in Red Wine and White Wine

ANTIOXIDANT COMPOUND	AVERAGE CONTENT (mg/liter)	
	RED WINE	WHITE WINE
Caffeic acid	7	3
Catechin	191	35
Cyanidin	3	0
Gallic acid	95	7
Myricetin	9	0
Rutin	82	21

Other scientists tested the antioxidant capacity of various red and white wines by measuring their ORAC scores (see Table 5.3).[5] The authors labeled any wine with a value over 1,230 as an "excellent" antioxidant.

TABLE 5.3. The Antioxidant Capacity of Some Red and White Wines

GRAPE VARIETAL, COUNTRY PRODUCED (WINERY)	ORAC VALUE (μTE/100 g)
RED WINES	
Cabernet sauvignon, Argentina	1,640
Cabernet sauvignon, France	2,120
Cabernet sauvignon, U.S. (Forest Glen Winery, CA)	1,140
Cabernet sauvignon, U.S. (Glen Ellen, CA)	1,010
Chambourcin, U.S. (Tomasello Winery, NJ)	1,470
Merlot, Argentina	1,710
Montepulciano, Italy	1,870
Tempranillo, Spain	1,890
Villard noir, U.S. (Atlantic County, NJ)	2,720
WHITE WINES	
Chardonnay, Italy	340
Chardonnay, U.S. (Mondavi Vineyards, CA)	420
Pinot grigio, Italy	290
Sauvignon blanc, France	260
Sauvignon blanc, U.S. (Woodbridge Winery, CA)	270
Vidal blanc (Mondavi Vineyards, CA)	330

As expected, after drinking red wine, the antioxidant capacity of the blood is increased.

In particular, the antioxidant resveratrol is found in abundance in grape skin. Its content in red wine is ap-

Grape skins, which are retained in the making of red wine, are loaded with antioxidants.

proximately twice its content in grape juice. In addition, certain antioxidant polyphenolic compounds are produced during the aging process of red wine. This means that although eating grapes may offer some benefits, drinking red wine is more beneficial. (White wine does contain the antioxidants hydroxytyrosol and tyrosol, which are capable of protecting the heart in a way similar to how the resveratrol in red wine does.[6])

Alcohol's Effects on Other Fruits

Strawberries and blackberries are naturally rich in oxidants, and treating them with alcohol boosts their antioxidant power, as reported by researchers in Thailand and by the USDA. Serving strawberries in daiquiri form may actually enhance their antioxidant capacity! Alternatively, storing strawberries and blackberries for a week or two in alcohol keeps them relatively fresh and prevents the decay of the antioxidants present in them.[7]

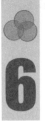

6

Antioxidant Vitamins and Minerals: To Supplement or Not?

Vitamins are probably the biggest-selling dietary supplements in the United States, where an estimated 35 percent of the population takes vitamin and mineral supplements. It is a multibillion dollar industry.[1] Vitamins are required by the body in very small amounts for growth and to maintain normal health. Because the human body cannot produce most vitamins on its own, we must get them from diet. The exceptions are vitamin K, which is produced by gut flora in the intestine, and vitamin D, which is synthesized when the skin is exposed to sunlight.

Vitamins are essential for the function of certain enzymes in the body and also important for other basic bodily functions. Some vitamins, as you know by now, are also antioxidants. Vitamins can be broadly classified into two categories: fat-soluble vitamins (vitamins A, D, E, and K) and water-soluble vitamins (vitamin B complex and C). Fat-soluble vitamins can be stored in the body; water-soluble vitamins cannot.

Minerals and trace elements are inorganic compounds that are essential for certain vital biochemical reactions in the human body. As mentioned in Chapter 1, selenium is the primary antioxidant mineral. Strictly speaking, selenium is not an antioxidant nutrient, but it is a component of antioxidant enzymes.

This chapter examines the risks and benefits of taking supplements of the antioxidant vitamins (C, A, and E) and of the antioxidant mineral selenium. It may also be useful for you to research the effects of supplementation of the other vitamins and minerals — i.e., those that do not have an antioxidant capacity — but such a discussion is beyond the scope of this book.

Vitamin C

Vitamin C (ascorbic acid), considered the most effective antioxidant vitamin, was the first vitamin supplement that was commercially available. One advantage of vitamin C is that it is water soluble, so excess vitamin C will be excreted in the urine without causing substantial toxicity. In contrast, vitamin E and beta-carotene are fat soluble, meaning excess intake of them may cause toxicity.

The beneficial effects of vitamin C were apparent long before its official discovery in 1932, because it was known for many years that eating citrus foods would prevent scurvy, a fatal disease that killed many sailors between 1500 and 1800. In the nineteenth century, British maritime law began requiring all ships to provide a daily ration of limes to each sailor to prevent scurvy (hence the nickname "limey" for British sailors, and then later for British immigrants to the colonies). Vitamin C plays many important roles in the body, including facilitating collagen formation. Collagen makes cartilage and other important tissues; lack of collagen synthesis is a major symptom of scurvy, leading to spots on the skin and bleeding from the gums and other mucus membranes.

In addition, the antioxidant effect of vitamin C has been well documented, leading researchers to speculate about the possible benefits of taking supplements of the vitamin. Diseases such as atherosclerosis (plaque formation in arteries that eventually may cause heart attack), stroke, and cancer may occur in part due to oxidative damage. Therefore, it can be hypothesized that vitamin C supplementation could prevent or lower the risk of such diseases. However, intervention studies failed to show any beneficial effect of vitamin C supplements in preventing disease or reducing oxidative stress.[2]

The daily requirement (RDA) of vitamin C can be easily fulfilled by a proper diet, and no vitamin C supplement is needed for a healthy person.

A single glass of orange juice or two oranges in the morning can provide almost all the vitamin C needed daily for a healthy person. However, be aware that vitamin C in orange juice may degrade if stored too long. Therefore, orange juice should be purchased at least three to four weeks before expiration and should be consumed within a week of purchase in order to get the highest intake of vitamin C.[3] Lemon juice, apple juice, and other fruit juices are also rich in vitamin C.

Professor Linus Pauling, two-time winner of the Nobel Prize, advocated in 1970 that intake of large doses of vitamin C could prevent colds, and scientists have been debating this issue ever since.[4] In one study, the authors analyzed data from twenty-nine different clinical trials involving 11,077 subjects and concluded that taking vitamin C at a dosage of 200 mg per day or more appears to reduce the severity and duration of colds but cannot prevent them from occurring.[5] Due to the failure of vitamin C to reduce incidence of the common cold in the normal population, I do not recommend taking regular megadoses of vitamin C (2–4 gm a day) in the hopes that you might avoid getting a cold.[6] There is no known benefit of high intake of vitamin C. In fact, excess vitamin C can exert various negative effects, including impaired absorption of iron.[7]

Beta-Carotene (Precursor to Vitamin A)

As mentioned previously, although vitamin A itself is found only in animal foods, its precursor, beta-carotene, is abundant in plants as the most common form of the pigment carotenoid. The RDA of vitamin A is 700 micrograms for women (0.7 milligrams or 2,310 IU) and 900 micrograms for men (0.9 milligrams or 3,000 IU). A daily intake of up to 3,000 micrograms (3 mg) of vitamin A is considered safe, but intake of excess vitamin A may cause toxicity, leading to higher risk of hip fracture and birth defects. Pregnant women should not consume excess vitamin A for this reason. Excess intake of vitamin A also interferes with absorption of vitamin D, causing deficiency of that vitamin. If the body has enough vitamin A then it does not make any vitamin A from beta-carotene, and excess carotene may turn the skin yellow.[8]

Because beta-carotene is a strong antioxidant numerous clinical trials have investigated whether its supplementation can prevent cancer and cardiovascular disease. Unfortunately, results from these trials showed no benefits of beta-carotene supplementation in preventing cancer or cardiovascular disease. In fact, supplementation (20–30 mg per day) could even increase the risk of lung and stomach cancer.[9] Moreover, a French study showed that even 2.1 mg daily supplementation with vitamin A may increase the risk of tobacco-related cancer. Therefore, the authors of the study recommended that the public be discouraged from taking beta-carotene supplements.[10] Sometimes the amount of beta-carotene or vitamin A is listed on package labels as IU. The conversion factor for IU of vitamin A to milligrams of beta-carotene is different from the conversion factor for vitamin E. For vitamin A, 1 IU equals 0.0006 milligrams of beta-carotene (or 0.6 micrograms).

Currently there is no evidence that taking supplements of carotenoids, including beta-carotene, offers any benefit.[11] Although it is not recommended that the general population take such supplements, under medical advice certain kinds of patients may benefit from them. For example, special eye vitamins are available for slowing down age-related macular degeneration (AMD) and other age-related eye diseases. These supplements contain antioxidant vitamins such as vitamins C, E, and beta-carotene, as well as the minerals zinc and copper.[12]

Vitamin E

Vitamin E exists in eight different forms, including alpha-, beta-, gamma-, and delta-tocopherol, as well as alpha-, beta-, gamma-, and delta-tocotrienol. Alpha-tocopherol is the most active form in humans.

Foods that contain vitamin E include eggs, fortified cereals, fruit, green leafy vegetables (such as spinach, avocado, almonds, asparagus, cucumber), meat, nuts/nut oils, poultry, vegetable oils (corn, cottonseed, safflower, soybean, sunflower, etc.). Some vitamin E may be destroyed during cooking and storage.

Vitamin E has been proposed for the prevention or treatment of numerous health conditions, often based on its antioxidant properties. Although older studies observed beneficial effects of vitamin E supplements in preventing heart disease, recent clinical trials failed to document any significant beneficial effect of vitamin E supplement in preventing *any* disease, not just heart disease. In contrast, taking excess vitamin E (400 IU per day or more) was found to be a health hazard: In clinical trials vitamin E increased mortality from all causes rather than reducing it.[13] A cancer-prevention study that looked at people who were already diagnosed with cancer concluded that vitamin E supplementation caused a 30 percent higher death rate![14]

> **No evidence exists from clinical trials that high-dose supplementation of vitamin E affords any health benefit. In fact, it may cause harm.**

Taking supplements rich in vitamin E may increase mortality because at higher dosages vitamin E may cause oxidative damage — acting as a pro-oxidant rather than an antioxidant.[15] Currently vitamin E should be taken under medical advice only by people who suffer from chronic vitamin E deficiency.[16]

Selenium

Selenium is an important antioxidant trace element found primarily in whole grains, shellfish, some nuts, and some meats (especially if the animal grazed on grass or grain grown in an area that has a high level of selenium in the soil). It helps in fighting infection, boosts sperm production in males, and may also afford some anticancer effect. Healthy adults need only 55 micrograms per day (60 for pregnant women and 70 for breastfeeding women). The upper tolerable limit is about 400 micrograms per day. Excess selenium is toxic (leading to selenosis) and may cause hair loss, brittle and discolored nails, nausea, diarrhea, and irritability. The soils of certain areas in the Great Plains and Western United States, as well as other parts of the world, contain high amounts of selenium, which is taken up by plants and thus found in the food supply. An outbreak of selenium poisoning is rare, but it does happen. Once, an outbreak of selenium toxicity occurred in ten different states in the United States, affecting 201 people who took liquid multivitamin supplements. The supplements contained 200 micrograms of selenium per ounce, according to the package insert, but actual analysis showed a selenium content 200 times higher than that. Although one person was hospitalized in this incident, no one died, and the company withdrew the faulty product from the market.[17] Excess selenium may also increase the risk of type 2 diabetes.[18]

RDAs and Tolerable Upper Limits: A Summary

Table 6.1 on the next page provides a quick summary of the RDAs and maximum tolerable limits of the three antioxidant vitamins and selenium.

Do You Need a Vitamin/ Mineral Supplement?

Currently there is no documented proof that taking multivitamin and mineral supplements can help prevent disease. Eating a balanced diet is the best way to fulfill your daily requirements of vitamins and minerals.

TABLE 6.1. The RDA and Tolerable Upper Limits for the Antioxidant Vitamins and Selenium

NUTRIENT	DEFICIENCY DISEASE	RDA	TOLERABLE UPPER INTAKE LIMIT (DAILY)
Vitamin A	Night blindness	900 µg, men 700 µg, women	3,000 µg
Vitamin C (ascorbic acid)	Scurvy, bleeding gums	90 mg, men 75 mg, women	2,000 mg
Vitamin E	Muscle fatigue, hair loss	15 mg	400 mg
Selenium	Heart disease, hypothyroidism, weakened immune system	55 µg	400 µg

Millions of postmenopausal women use multivitamins, often believing that supplements prevent chronic diseases such as cancer and cardiovascular disease, but no convincing evidence supports the notion that multivitamin supplements prevent any disease in postmenopausal women.[19] Furthermore, some researchers have concluded that beta-carotene and vitamin E supplements, in particular, may cause more harm than good.[20] Healthy people eating a balanced diet every day do not require any supplements. However, pregnant women should take a multivitamin, along with folate and iron supplements, and elderly people may benefit from vitamin supplements. My recommendation is to take vitamin and mineral supplements only when recommended by your doctor.

Other Antioxidant Supplements

The popularity of herbal supplements is steadily increasing among the general population in the United States. It is estimated that approximately one out of five adults has used an herbal supplement within the past year. The laws governing dietary supplements in the United States make it illegal for a manufacturer to claim any medical benefits for a supplement. Unfortunately, the FDA (Food and Drug Administration) does not have authority to stop a supplement from being marketed, even if research indicates it is unsafe. In 2002 the FDA issued a warning regarding the safety of kava, an herbal sedative often used to reduce anxiety. Prolonged use of kava can cause liver damage serious enough to require liver transplant or even to cause death. Yet kava is still available from some health-food stores. By contrast, in Germany, government-sanctioned publications (monographs) exist recommending certain supplements for treating specific conditions. If an herb is unsafe to use then there is no monograph on it. Currently, there is a push in the European Union to standardize rules for marketing herbal supplements. In Canada, the federal government has implemented a policy to regulate natural health products.[1]

Sales of herbal supplements are not regulated by the FDA in the United States.

The ten most commonly used herbal supplements, in order, are echinacea, ginseng, ginkgo biloba, garlic, St. John's wort, peppermint, ginger, soy, chamomile, and kava.[2]

To my knowledge no studies exist addressing the benefits or dangers of taking an antioxidant herbal supplement in healthy people. My recommendation is to avoid taking antioxidant herbal supplements if you are healthy. Instead, focus your efforts on eating a balanced diet, with plenty of antioxidant-rich fruits and vegetables, every day. Sometimes, herbal supplements may be useful in treating certain medical conditions. If you wish to take any supplement for treating a condition, I recommend that you talk to your doctor first.

Healthy people eating a balanced diet every day, including at least five servings of antioxidant-rich vegetables and fruits, do not need to take dietary supplements on a regular basis.

The rest of this chapter summarizes the effects of antioxidant herbal (plant-based) supplements and other supplements that have antioxidant properties. If you're interested in reading about supplements that are not antioxidant in nature, there are excellent books on the safety and efficacy of herbal supplements, including my first book on consumer health, *Prescription or Poison? The Benefits and Dangers of Herbal Remedies* (Hunter House, 2010).

Antioxidant Herbal Supplements

Because plants are rich in antioxidants, it may seem obvious to assume that many herbal supplements are also rich in antioxidants. Unfortunately, papers published in medical literature describe relatively few herbs with antioxidant properties. Table 7.1 lists the most common antioxidant herbal supplements and their uses.

TABLE 7.1. Common Antioxidant Herbal Supplements

(Primary Indications Appear in **Bold**; Possible Contraindications [Indications Against Use] and Interactions with Other Drugs Appear in *Italics*)

SUPPLEMENT	INDICATIONS FOR USE
Astragalus	**Boosting immune function** (thus helping to prevent common cold); anticancer properties; used in China to treat heart disease (raises good cholesterol/lowers bad cholesterol)
Berry extracts (general effects; see individual listings that follow for specific effects)	**Anticancer properties; protection from heart disease (prevention of plaque buildup in arteries);** possible treatment for diabetes; improvement in night vision; protection against memory loss in the elderly
Bilberry extract	**Improving circulation;** treating diarrhea and menstrual cramps

(cont'd.)

**TABLE 7.1. Common Antioxidant Herbal Supplements
(cont'd.)**

SUPPLEMENT	INDICATIONS FOR USE
Blueberry extract	**Improving circulation**
Cat's claw	**Preventing inflammation/osteoarthritis;** boosting immune system; treating cancer; treating arthritis; preventing pregnancy; *should be avoided during pregnancy or when trying to become pregnant*
Chaste berry extract	**Treating menstrual problems,** including related breast pain (mastalgia); treating menopausal symptoms; *should be avoided during pregnancy and lactation*
Cranberry extract	**Preventing urinary tract infection;** possible prevention of kidney stones; may have action against the bacterium that causes the majority of stomach ulcers (*H. pylori*); may improve cholesterol levels in diabetics
Elderberry extract	**Treating cold and flu**
Garlic extract	**Lowering blood cholesterol and triglycerides;** preventing heart attack and stroke; preventing cancer; reducing risk of dementia in the elderly; *should be avoided by patients taking a blood thinner such as warfarin (but using garlic as a spice in reasonable amounts is safe for everyone)*
Ginkgo biloba	**Sharpening memory** (clinical results show varied effects); *should be avoided by patients taking a blood thinner such as warfarin*

(cont'd.)

TABLE 7.1. Common Antioxidant Herbal Supplements (cont'd.)

SUPPLEMENT	INDICATIONS FOR USE
Ginseng, including Asian ginseng (*Panax ginseng*), American ginseng (*Panax quinquefolius*), and Siberian ginseng (*Eleutherococcus senticosus*)	**Tonic for good health; lowering blood sugar;** anticancer properties; anti-inflammatory agent; improvement in performance and memory; possible treatment for insomnia; *should be avoided by patients taking a blood thinner such as warfarin*
Grapeseed extract	**Reducing risk of blocked coronary arteries; lowering cholesterol;** reducing complications of diabetes; preventing cancer; wound healing
Lycopene supplement	**Preventing cardiovascular disease; preventing certain cancers** (clinical studies show conflicting results for cancer prevention)
Milk thistle	**Treating liver problems;** treating viral infection; possible anticancer, antidiabetic, and cholesterol-lowering effects
Soy supplement	**Weight reduction; lowering cholesterol; relief from symptoms of menopause;** reducing risk of breast cancer; treating osteoporosis
St. John's wort	**Antidepressant;** treating anxiety and sleep disorders; possible antibacterial, anti-inflammatory, and antitumor properties; *see Table 7.2 on the next page for a list of prescription drugs whose effectiveness may be seriously compromised if taken with St. John's wort, possibly leading to treatment failure*

(cont'd.)

TABLE 7.1. Common Antioxidant Herbal Supplements (cont'd.)

SUPPLEMENT	INDICATIONS FOR USE
Turmeric	**Treating digestive problems; treating arthritis (including rheumatoid arthritis);** antibacterial, antiviral, antifungal, antioxidant, anticancer properties; possible protection against Alzheimer's disease; treatment of other chronic illnesses

St. John's wort can interfere with many prescription drugs. Patients receiving warfarin therapy, transplant recipients, and patients being treated for AIDS may face serious treatment failure if they start taking St. John's wort. Major interactions between Western drugs and St. John's wort are listed in Table 7.2.

> If you are taking any medications on a regular basis for treating any chronic health problem, do not take St. John's wort without approval from your physician.

TABLE 7.2. Common Drug Interactions with St. John's Wort, Leading to Potential Treatment Failure

CLASS OF MEDICATION	NAME OF DRUG
Antiasthmatic agent	Theophylline
Anticancer agents	Imatinib, irinotecan
Anticoagulant agent (blood thinner)	Warfarin
Antidepressant	Amitriptyline
Antiepileptics (seizure control)	Phenobarbital, phenytoin

(cont'd.)

TABLE 7.2. Common Drug Interactions with St. John's Wort, Leading to Potential Treatment Failure (cont'd.)

CLASS OF MEDICATION	NAME OF DRUG
Anti-inflammatory agent	Ibuprofen
Antimicrobial agents (antibiotic/antifungal)	Erythromycin, voriconazole
Anti-Parkinson's agent	Levodopa
Antiretroviral agents (used for treating AIDS)	Atazanavir, indinavir, lamivudine, nevirapine, saquinavir
Benzodiazepines (sedative/anti-anxiety)	Alprazolam, midazolam
Cardioactive agents	Digoxin, nifedipine, verapamil
Hypoglycemic agents (used to lower blood sugar)	Gliclazide, tolbutamide
Immunosuppressive agents (used in transplant patients to prevent organ rejection)	Cyclosporine, tacrolimus
Oral contraceptives	Ethinyl estradiol and other formulas
Proton pump inhibitor (used in treating acid reflux)	Omeprazole
Statins (used to lower blood cholesterol)	Atorvastatin, pravastatin
Synthetic opioid (used in drug rehabilitation)	Methadone

Other (Nonherbal) Antioxidant Supplements

In addition to antioxidant herbs, a few other supplements typically sold in health-food stores have significant antioxidant activities. These supplements are listed in Table 7.3 on the next page.

TABLE 7.3. Common Nonherbal Antioxidant Supplements

(Primary Indications Appear in **Bold**; Possible Contraindications and Interactions with Other Drugs Appear in *Italics*)

SUPPLEMENT	INDICATIONS FOR USE
Alpha-lipoic acid	**Preventing complications of diabetes;** may improve vision
Coenzyme Q10 (CoQ10)	**Preventing heart disease and heart failure; treating high blood pressure; increasing energy;** possible adjunct therapy for Parkinson's disease; *may interact with many drugs such as the anticoagulant warfarin, cholesterol-lowering drugs, diabetic medicines, antidepressants, and others*
Glucosamine (alone or in combination with chondroitin)	**Treating osteoarthritis**
Glutathione (oral)	**General antioxidant effects** (clinical trial showed mixed results)
Melatonin	**Correcting sleep-wake cycle;** improving immune function

Even though antioxidant supplements may be effective, healthy individuals probably don't need them to boost their antioxidant defense. As I've stated elsewhere, eating a balanced diet every day is sufficient to ensure adequate antioxidant defense in a healthy person. However, under certain disease conditions taking supplements may be useful. I strongly recommend you to talk to your doctor before taking any antioxidant supplements.

Conclusion

I hope this book has fulfilled its primary aim: demonstrating both the importance of boosting your body's natural antioxidant defense and the relative ease of doing so by eating a well-balanced diet rich in fruits and vegetables. No matter the state of your health, you will benefit by following the dietary recommendations presented here. If you have specific health complaints or concerns, consult with a nutritionally minded doctor to decide whether additional antioxidant support in the form of supplements would be right for you.

Remember that knowledge is power. The goal of this book is to empower you to make decisions that will help you achieve the best health possible.

If you would like to contact me, please e-mail me at amitava.dasgupta@uth.tmc.edu.

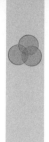

Notes

Chapter 1

1. USDA website, http://www.ars.usda.gov/services/docs.htm ?docid=15866 (accessed October 2012).
2. R. L. Prior, "Antioxidant Food Databases: Valuable or Not?" http://www.brunswicklabs.com/Portals/153979/docs/A%20 Response%20to%20the%20USDA%20ORAC%20Statement .pdf (accessed October 2012).

Chapter 2

1. F. L. Crowe et al., "Fruit and Vegetable Intake and Mortality from Ischaemic Heart Disease: Results from the European Prospective Investigation into Cancer and Nutrition (EPIC)-Heart Study," *European Heart Journal* 32 (2011): 1235–43.
2. P. M. Kris-Etherton, W. S. Harris, and L. J. Apple, "Fish Consumption, Fish Oil, Omega-3-Fatty Acids and Cardiovascular Disease," *Circulation* 106 (2002): 2747–57.
3. I. Afanas'ev, "Reactive Oxygen Species Signalling in Cancer: Comparison with Aging," *Aging and Disease* 2, no. 3 (2011): 219–30.

Chapter 3

1. J. W. Finley et al., "Antioxidants in Foods: State of the Science Important to the Food Industry," *Journal of Agricultural Food Chemistry* 59 (2011): 6837–46.
2. B. L. Halvorsen et al., "Content of Redox-Active Compounds (i.e., Antioxidants) in Foods Consumed in the United States," *American Journal of Clinical Nutrition* 84 (2006): 95–135.

3. L. M. McCune et al., "Cherries and Health: A Review," *Critical Review of Food Science and Nutrition* 51 (2011): 1–12.

4. S. U. Mertens-Talcott et al., "Pharmacokinetics of Anthocyanins and Antioxidant Effects After the Consumption of Anthocyanin-Rich Açai Juice and Pulp (*Euterpe oleracea Mart.*) in Human Healthy Volunteers," *Journal of Agricultural Food Chemistry* 56 (2008): 7796–7802.

5. R. G. Ziegler et al., "Carotenoid Intake, Vegetables and the Risk of Lung Cancer Among White Men in New Jersey," *American Journal of Epidemiology* 123 (1986): 1080–93.

6. C. Dincer et al., "Effects of Baking and Boiling on the Nutritional and Antioxidant Properties of Sweet Potato [*Ipomea batatas (L)Lam*] Cultivates," *Plant Food and Human Nutrition* 66 (2011): 341–47.

7. C. M. Kaefer and J. A. Milner, "The Role of Herbs and Spices in Cancer Prevention," *Journal of Nutrition and Biochemistry* 19 (2008): 347–61.

8. J. Gruenwald, J. Freder, and N. Armbruster, "Cinnamon and Health," *Critical Review of Food Science and Nutrition* 50 (2010): 822–34.

9. A. Iyer et al., "Potential Health Benefits of Indian Spices in the Symptoms of the Metabolic Syndrome: A Review," *Indian Journal of Biochemistry and Biophysics* 46 (2009): 467–81.

10. R. Blomhoff et al., "Health Benefits of Nuts: Potential Role of Antioxidants," *British Journal of Nutrition* 96, suppl. 2 (2008): S52–60.

11. P. M. Kris-Etherton, F. B. Hu, and J. Sabete, "The Role of Tree Nuts and Peanuts in the Prevention of Coronary Heart Disease: Multiple Potential Mechanisms," *Journal of Nutrition* 138 (2008): 1746S–1751S.

12. J. A. Vinson and Y. Cai, "Nuts, Especially Walnuts, Have Both Antioxidant Quantity and Efficacy and Exhibit Significant Potential Health Benefits," *Food and Function* 3 (2012): 134–40.

13. E. Hallmann and E. Rembialkowska, "Characterisation of Antioxidant Compounds in Sweet Bell Pepper (*Capsicum annuum L.*) Under Organic and Conventional Growing

Systems," *Journal of the Science of Food and Agriculture* 92(2012):2409–2415

14. E. Hallmann, "The Influence of Organic and Conventional Cultivation Systems on the Nutritional Value and Content of Bioactive Compounds in Selected Tomato Types," *Journal of the Science of Food and Agriculture* Feb 20, 2012 [e-pub ahead of print].

15. D. Hunter et al., "Evaluation of the Micronutrients Composition of Plant Foods Produced by Organic and Conventional Agricultural Methods," *Critical Review of Food and Nutrition* 51 (2011): 571–82.

16. M. D. Raigon, A. Rodriguez-Burruezo, and J. Prohens, "Effects of Organic and Conventional Cultivation Methods on Composition of Eggplant Fruits," *Journal of Agricultural Food Chemistry* 58 (2010): 6833–40.

17. P. Juroszek et al., "Fruit Quality and Bioactive Compounds with Antioxidant Activity of Tomatoes Grown on Farm: Comparison of Organic and Conventional Management System," *Journal of Agricultural Food Chemistry* 57 (2009): 1188–94.

Chapter 4

1. J. Bonita et al., "Coffee and Cardiovascular Disease: In Vitro, Cellular, Animal and Human Studies," *Pharmacological Research* 55(2007): 187–98.

2. F. Natella et al., "Coffee Drinking Influences Plasma Antioxidant Capacity in Humans," *Journal of Agricultural Food Chemistry* 50 (2002): 6211–66.

3. E. W. Chan et al., "Antioxidant and Antibacterial Properties of Green, Black and Herbal Teas of *Camellia sinensis,*" *Pharmacognosy Research* 3(2011): 266–72.

4. J. V. Higdon and B. Frei, "Coffee and Health: A Review of Recent Human Research," *Critical Review in Food Science and Nutrition* 46 (2006): 101–123.

Chapter 5

1. R. Dudley, "Ethanol, Fruit Ripening and the Historical Ori-

gins of Human Alcoholism in Primate Frugivory," *Integrative and Comparative Biology* 44, no 4 (August 2004): 315–23.

2. United States Department of Agriculture and United States Department of Health and Human Services, *Dietary Guidelines for Americans,* "Chapter 9: Alcoholic Beverages" (Washington, DC: US Government Printing Office, 2005), 43–46, http://www.health.gov/DIETARYGUIDELINES/dga 2005/document/html/chapter9.htm (accessed October 6, 2010).

3. A. Britton and M. Marmot, "Different Measures of Alcohol Consumption and Risk of Coronary Heart Disease and All Cause Mortality: A 11 Year Follow Up of the Whitehall II Cohort Study," *Addiction* 99, no 1 (January 2004): 109–116.

4. G. J. Soleas, E. P. Diamandis, and D. M. Goldberg, "Wine As a Biological Fluid: History, Production and Role in Disease Prevention," *Journal of Clinical Laboratory Analysis*11, no 5 (September 1997): 287–313.

5. C. Sanchez-Moreno et al., "Anthocyanin and Proanthocyanidin Content in Selected White Wine and Red Wines. Oxygen Radical Absorbance Capacity Comparison with Nontraditional Wines Obtained from Highbush Blueberry," *Journal of Agricultural and Food Chemistry* 51, no 17 (August 2003): 4889–96.

6. J. I. Dudley et al., "Does White Wine Qualify for French Paradox? Comparison of Cardioprotective Effects of Red and White Wines and Their Constituents: Resveratrol, Tyrosol and Hydroxytyrosol," *Journal of Agricultural and Food Chemistry* 56, no 20 (October 2008): 9362–73.

7. K. Chanjirakul et al., "Natural Volatile Treatments Increase Free-Radical Scavenging Capacity of Strawberries and Blackberries," *Journal of the Science of Food and Agriculture* 87 (2007): 1463–72.

Chapter 6

1. C. L. Rock, "Multivitamin-Multi-Mineral Supplements: Who Uses Them?" *American Journal of Clinical Nutrition* 85 (2007): 277S–279S.

2. V. S. Talaulikar and I. T. Manyonda, "Vitamin C as an Anti-oxidant Supplement in Women's Health: A Myth in Need of Urgent Burial," *European Journal of Obstetrics Gynecology and Reproductive Biology* 157 (2011): 10–13.

3. C. S. Johnston and D. L. Bowling, "Stability of Ascorbic Acid in Commercially Available Orange Juices," *Journal of the American Dietetic Association* 102 (2002): 525–29.

4. H. Hemilä, "Vitamin C Supplementation and the Common Cold — Was Linus Pauling Right or Wrong?" *International Journal of Vitamin and Nutrition Research* 67 (1997): 329–35.

5. R. M. Douglas and H. Hemilä, "Vitamin C for Preventing and Treating the Common Cold," *Cochrane Database Systematic Review* 4 (2004): CD000980.

6. R. M. Douglas et al., "Vitamin C for Preventing and Treating the Common Cold," *Cochrane Database Systematic Review* 3 (2007): CD000980.

7. T. W. Anderson, "Large Scale Studies with Vitamin C," *Acta Vitaminologica et Enzymologica* 31 (1977): 43–50.

8. K. L. Penniston and S. A. Tanumihardjo, "The Acute and Chronic Toxic Effects of Vitamin A," *American Journal of Clinical Nutrition* 71 (2006): 1325S–33S.

9. N. Druesne-Pecollo et al., "Beta-Carotene Supplementation and Cancer Risk: A Systematic Review and Metaanalysis of Randomized Controlled Trials," *International Journal of Cancer* 127 (2010): 172–84.

10. T. Tanvetyanon and G. Bepler, "Beta-Carotene in Multivitamins and the Possible Risk of Lung Cancer Among Smokers Versus Former Smokers: A Meta Analysis and Evaluation of National Brands," *Cancer* 113 (2008): 150–57.

11. S. Voutilainen et al., "Carotenoids and Cardiovascular Health," *American Journal of Clinical Nutrition* 83 (2006): 1265–71.

12. H. P. Sin, D. T. Liu, and D. S. Lam, "Lifestyle Modification, Nutritional and Vitamins Supplements for Age Related Macular Degeneration," *Acta Ophthalmologica* 2012 [e-pub ahead of print].

13. H. Y. Huang et al., "The Efficacy and Safety of Multivitamin and Mineral Supplement Use to Prevent Cancer and Chronic Disease in Adults: A Systematic Review for a National Institutes of Health State of the Science Conference." *Annals of Internal Medicine* 145 (2006): 372–85.

14. M. G. Soni et al., "Safety of Vitamins and Minerals: Controversies and Perspective," *Toxicological Sciences* 118 (2010): 348–55.

15. Ibid.

16. Y. Dotan, D. Lichtenberg, and I. Pinchuk, "No Evidence Supports Vitamin E Indiscriminate Supplementation," *Biofactors* 35 (2009): 469–73.

17. J. K. MacFarquhar et al., "Acute Selenium Toxicity Associated with a Dietary Supplement," *Archives of Internal Medicine* 170 (2010): 256–71.

18. J. Bleys, A. Navas-Acien, and E. Guallar, "Serum Selenium and Diabetes in U.S. Adults," *Diabetes Care* 30 (2007): 829–34.

19. M. L. Neuhouser et al., "Multivitamin Use and Risk of Cancer and Cardiovascular Disease in Women's Health Initiative Cohorts," *Archives of Internal Medicine* 169 (2009): 294–304.

20. G. Bjelakovic et al., "Antioxidant Supplements for Prevention of Mortality in Healthy Participants and Patients with Various Diseases," *Cochrane Database Systematic Review* 14 (2012): 3: CD 007176.

Chapter 7

1. K. Moss et al., "New Canadian Natural Health Product Regulations: A Qualitative Study on How CAM Practitioners Perceive They Will Be Impacted," *BMC Complementary and Alternative Medicine* 10, no. 6 (2006):18.

2. S. Bent, "Herbal Medicine in the United States: Review of Efficacy, Safety and Regulation," *Journal of General Internal Medicine* 23 (2008): 854–59.

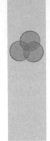

Resources

Websites

www.oracvalues.com: Provides a database compiled by the National Institute on Aging of the National Institutes of Health (NIH) that includes measurements of antioxidant levels in foods.

www.livestrong.com: Provides links to many informative articles on antioxidants.

www.nlm.nih.gov/medlineplus: A database within the National Institute of Health's website that includes information on antioxidants.

http://usda.gov: Provides a list of links to online articles on antioxidants by the United States Department of Agriculture.

Books

Kinderlehrer, Daniel A., and Janet Kinderlehrer. *The Antioxidant Save-Your-Life Cookbook: 150 Nutritious, High-Fiber, Low-Fat Recipes to Protect You Against the Damaging Effects of Free Radicals*. New York: Newmarket Press, 2007.

Moss, Ralph W. *Antioxidants Against Cancer*. New York: Equinox Press, 1999.

Passwater, Richard. *The Antioxidants*. New Canaan, CT: Keats Publishing, Inc., 1985.

Stewart Riccio, Dolores. *Antioxidant Power: 366 Delicious Recipes for Great Health and Long Life*. New York: Plume, 1999.

Weiner, Michael. *The Antioxidant Cookbook: A Nutritionist's Secret Strategy*. Nashville, TN: Hambleton-Hill, 1996.

Yoshikawa, T., L. Packer, and M. Hiramatsu, eds. *Antioxidant Food Supplements in Human Health*. San Diego, CA: Academic Press, 1999.

Index

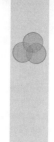

Figures and tables are indicated with *f* and *t* following the page number.

A

açai berries, 45–46
acetaminophen, 24
air pollution, 5
alcohol, 10, 67–73, 70*t*, 71*t*, 72*t*
alpha-lipoic acid (ALA), 11, 90
amino acids, 3
anthocyanins, 32, 44
antioxidants, overview: classes and compounds of, 32*t*; definition and function, 10; tests measuring capacity levels of, 12–14; tests measuring food's content of, 39; types and dietary sources of, 11–12. *See also related topics*
anxiety, 5, 20
astaxanthin, 29–30
astragalus, 85

B

bell peppers, 53–54
berries, 44–45, 45*t*, 73
berry extracts, 85
beta-carotene: dietary sources of, 30, 36*t*, 49; as exogenous antioxidant, 11, 12; recommended dietary allowance, 35, 77; supplementation benefits and risks, 28, 77–79, 81; tests measuring levels of, 14; vitamin A conversion, 33, 35
beta-cryptoxanthin, 30
bilberry extract, 85
blood pressure, 27, 28*f*, 63
blueberry extract, 86
breakfast cereals, 55

C

cafestol, 57
caffeic acid, 31, 57
caffeine, 31, 56, 60–61, 62–63
cancer: diet reducing risk of, 27, 28*f*, 48; and oxidative stress, 21–22, 21*f*; supplementation increasing risks of, 78, 79–80
capsaicin, 31, 32
carbohydrates, 3
cardiovascular (heart) diseases: diet reducing risk of, 19–20, 19*t*, 28*f*; factors contributing to risk of, 20; foods and beverages reducing risk of, 65, 69, 70; and oxidative stress, 17–21; and vitamin E supplementation research, 79

carotenoids, 12, 29–30, 32, 49
catalase, 11
catechins, 57, 64
cat's claw, 86
chaste berry extract, 86
chemicals, household, 7–9t
cherries, 45
children, 20
chlorogenic acid, 57
chocolate, 56, 63–66, 64t
cholesterol, 18, 51, 53, 57
chondroitin, 90
cinnamon, 51
coenzyme Q10 (CoQ10), 11, 90
coffee, 31, 56–58, 58t, 60–63
cooking, effects of, 39, 41t, 42, 48
cranberry extract, 86
curcumin, 31

D
depression, 5, 19, 20
diabetes, 18, 22–23, 24f, 27, 28f, 81
diet: and cardiovascular health,
    19–20, 19t; recommendations,
    27, 28, 84; supplementation
    vs., 84, 90
diseases: alcohol consumption
    and risk of, 68; causing oxi-
    dative stress, overview, 15–16;
    diet as prevention strategy, 81;
    supplementation increasing
    risk of, 28, 78, 79–80; supple-
    mentation reducing risk of,
    76, 77, 81–82. See also specific
    names of diseases
DNA, 3, 21, 21f
drugs, 9–10t, 18, 24, 88–89t

E
eggplant, 54
elderberry extract, 86
endogenous antioxidants, 11

epicatechins, 64
exogenous antioxidants, 11–12

F
FDA (Food and Drug Adminis-
    tration), 83
fish, 19, 20, 38t, 55
flavonoids, 30, 32t, 65
foods: antioxidant-rich, ratings
    of, 40t; cooking affecting
    antioxidant contents of,
    39, 41t, 42; tests measuring
    antioxidants in, 12–14. See
    also diet; specific types of foods
FRAP (ferric-reducing ability
    of plasma) tests, 39
free radicals, 2–4, 16–17, 24
fruit juices, 47t, 76–77
fruits: antioxidant-rich, 40t,
    44–46, 45t, 46–47t; antioxi-
    dants in, 28–31; beta-caro-
    tene content of, 36t; and
    cardiovascular health, 19, 20;
    cooking affecting antioxidant
    content of, 41t; health benefits
    of, 27, 28f; ORAC value
    recommendations, 42–44;
    recommended daily servings,
    55; skins of, 46; vitamin E
    content of, 38t

G
garlic extract, 86
ginkgo biloba, 86
ginseng, 87
glucosamine, 90
glucose 6-phosphate deficiency,
    9
glutathione, 11, 14, 90
grains, 28f, 55
grapeseed extract, 87
grief, 5

H

Halvorsen, B. L., 37, 39
heart diseases. *See* cardiovascular (heart) diseases
herbal supplements, 83–89, 85–88*t*, 88–89*t*
herbs, 51, 52*t*
hydroxytyrosol, 73
hyperglycemia, 23

I

industrial pollution, 5
industrial solvents, 5
inflammation, 25–26
insulin, 22, 23, 51
insulin resistance, 22–23
isoflavones, 32

K

kahweol, 57
kidney disease, 23–25

L

lipids, 3
lutein, 11, 12, 30, 49
lycopene, 11, 12, 30, 49, 87

M

meat, 55
medications, 9–10*t*, 88–89*t*
melatonin, 90
mercury, 20
microwave cooking, 41*t*
milk thistle, 87
minerals, 74–75, 80–82, 82*t*

N

nucleic acids, 3
nuts, 28*f*, 42–43, 53, 54*t*

O

oils, 38*t*

ORAC (oxygen radical absorbance capacity) values: of chocolate, 64*t*; of coffee and tea, 58*t*; of fruits and fruit juices, 44–46, 45*t*, 46–47*t*; of herbs and spices, 51, 52*t*; of nuts, 53, 54*t*; overview and testing values, 12–14, 42, 45*t*, 46–47*t*; recommended values, 42–43; serving sizes and, 43; of vegetables, 49–51*t*; of wine, 72*t*
organic *vs.* conventional foods, 53–55
oxidation, 1, 2
oxidative stress: alcohol consumption contributing to, 69; definition and cause, 1, 2; diseases linked to, 15–17, 20–26, 21*f*; factors contributing to, 4–10*t*; tests measuring, 14; vitamin supplementation reducing risk of, 76

P

pain relievers, 10, 24
Pauling, Linus, 77
peanuts, 53
phenolic acids and esters, 30, 32
phytochemicals, 28, 30–31, 54
pollution, 5
polyphenols, 30–31, 57
polyunsaturated fatty acids, 3
pregnancy, 20, 62, 63, 69, 78, 82
Prior, Ronald, 13
proanthocyanidins, 64

R

radiation, 6
recommended dietary allowances (RDAs), 31, 33, 35, 37, 77, 82*t*

reduction, 1
restaurant dining, 55
resveratrol, 31, 32, 72–73

S
selenium, 11, 80–81, 82*t*
soy supplements, 87
spices, 51, 52*t*
St. John's wort, 87, 88–89*t*
stilbenoids, 30, 32
stress, 5, 18, 20. *See also* oxidative stress
sunlight, 6
superoxide dismutase (SOD), 11
supplements: government regulations of, 83–84; herbal, 37, 83–90, 85–88*t*, 88–89*t*; other, 89–90, 90*t*; vitamins and minerals, 28, 74–82, 82*t*
sweet potatoes, 48

T
tea, 56, 58–60, 58*t*, 62, 63
thearubigin, 57
theobromine, 56
tobacco smoking, 6
tomatoes, 54
turmeric, 88
Tylenol, 24
tyrosol, 73

V
vegetables: antioxidant-rich, 40*t*, 48–51*t*; antioxidants in, 28–31; beta-carotene content of, 36*t*; and cardiovascular health, 19, 20; cooking affecting antioxidant content of, 41*t*; health benefits of, 27, 28*f*; ORAC value recommendations, 42–44; recommended daily servings, 55; vitamin E content of, 38*t*
vitamin A, 11, 29, 33, 35, 82*t*. *See also* beta-carotene
vitamin C: dietary sources of, 29, 76–77; as exogenous antioxidant, 11, 14; recommended dietary allowance of, 33, 76, 82*t*; storage and stability, 33; supplementation risks and benefits, 75–77
vitamin D, 74, 78
vitamin E: dietary sources of, 29, 35, 37, 38*t*, 79; as exogenous antioxidant, 11, 14; forms of, 79; function of, 35; recommended dietary allowance, 37, 82*t*; supplementation risks and benefits, 28, 79–80, 82
vitamins: as antioxidants, 11, 14, 74; categories of, 74; supplementation of, 74–80, 81–82, 82*t*. *See also specific vitamins*

W
wine, 67, 69, 71–73, 71*t*, 72*t*. *See also* alcohol

X
xanthophylls, 49

Z
zeaxanthin, 30